This book is dedicated to my family, friends, and loved ones who have been with me from the very beginning. Without all of you I would not be where I am today.

Thank you to Stephen, Tyler, and Patricia, my editorial, design, and production team for your guidance, support, and most of all friendship.

Special thanks to my cousin, Bethany, for guiding me throughout my initial journeys with psychedelics, as well as countless others who have supported our team during the creation of this book.

Cooking with Magic Mushrooms: The Psilocybin Cookbook

This is Microcosm #833
ISBN 9781648413124
Illustrated by Snowflake

With a Safety Introduction by Erica Darragh

Photographs by Fractal Lion

First Edition, September 17, 2024
Cover and Book Design by Joe Biel

Microcosm Publishing
2752 N Williams Ave
Portland, OR 97227
(503)799-2698
Write or visit for a catalog
All the news that's fit to print at www.Microcosm.Pub/Newsletter

Get more copies of this book at www.Microcosm.Pub/MagicMushrooms

Find more resources about mushrooms at www.Microcosm.pub/Mushrooms

To join the ranks of high-class stores that feature Microcosm titles, talk to your rep: In the U.S. **COMO** (Atlantic), **ABRAHAM** (Midwest), **BOB BARNETT** (Texas, Oklahoma, Arkansas, Louisiana), **IMPRINT** (Pacific), **TURNAROUND** (UK), **UTP/MANDA** (Canada), **NEWSOUTH** (Australia/New Zealand), **Observatoire** (Africa, Europe), **IPR** (Middle East), **Yvonne Chau** (Southeast Asia), **HarperCollins** (India), **Everest/B.K. Agency** (China), **Tim Burland** (Japan/Korea), and **FAIRE** in the gift trade.

Global labor conditions are bad, and our roots in industrial Cleveland in the 70s and 80s made us appreciate the need to treat workers right. Therefore, our books are MADE IN THE USA.

Library of Congress Cataloging-in-Publication Data

Names: Connell, David, 1988- author.
Title: Cooking with magic mushrooms : the psilocybin cookbook / by David Connell (author).
Description: Portland : Microcosm Publishing, [2024] | Summary: "Magic mushrooms offer so many marvels, from transformative healing to excitement. One thing they are not known for is flavor. David Connell's quest to make psilocybin palatable led him to develop recipes that integrate small, measured quantities of shrooms into tasty food and drink"-- Provided by publisher.
Identifiers: LCCN 2024023018 | ISBN 9781648413124 (paperback)
Subjects: LCSH: Cooking (Mushrooms) | Mushrooms, Hallucinogenic. | Psilocybin--Therapeutic use. | Depression, Mental--Treatment--Popular works. | LCGFT: Cookbooks.
Classification: LCC TX804 .C66 2024 | DDC 641.6/58--dc23/eng/20240617
LC record available at https://lccn.loc.gov/2024023018

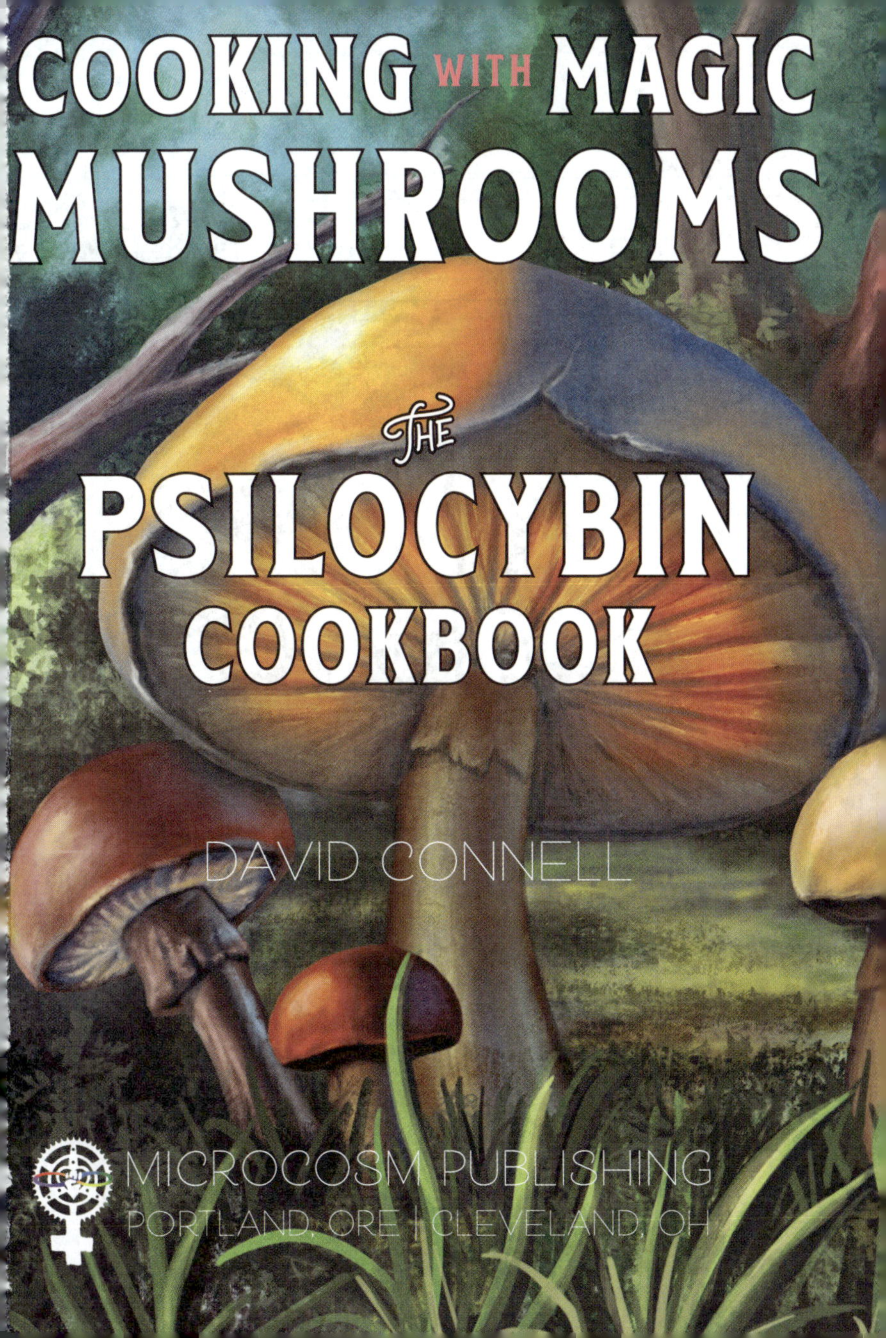

COOKING WITH MAGIC MUSHROOMS

THE PSILOCYBIN COOKBOOK

DAVID CONNELL

MICROCOSM PUBLISHING
PORTLAND, ORE | CLEVELAND, OH

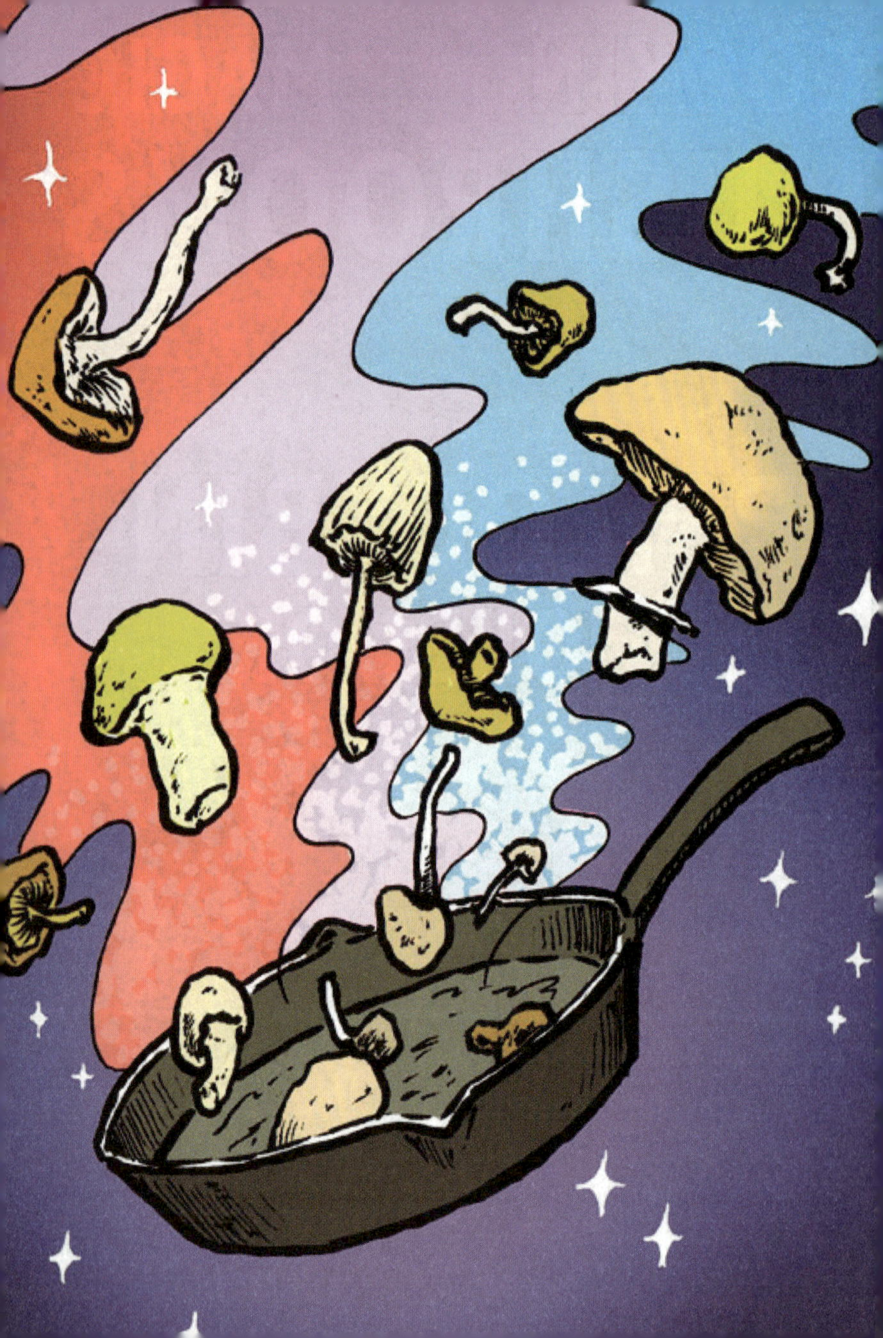

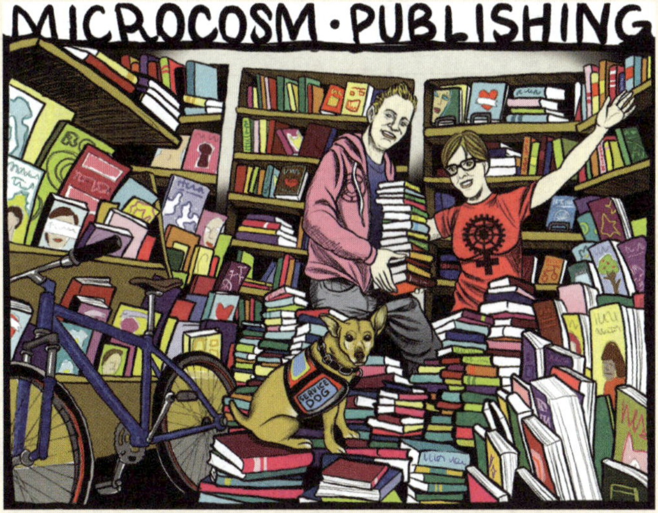

MICROCOSM PUBLISHING is Portland's most diversified publishing house and distributor, with a focus on the colorful, authentic, and empowering. Our books and zines have put your power in your hands since 1996, equipping readers to make positive changes in their lives and in the world around them. Microcosm emphasizes skill-building, showing hidden histories, and fostering creativity through challenging conventional publishing wisdom with books and bookettes about DIY skills, food, bicycling, gender, self-care, and social justice. What was once a distro and record label started by Joe Biel in a drafty bedroom was determined to be *Publishers Weekly*'s fastest-growing publisher of 2022 and #3 in 2023 and 2024, and is now among the oldest independent publishing houses in Portland, OR, and Cleveland, OH. We are a politically moderate, centrist publisher in a world that has inched to the right for the past 80 years.

Did you know that you can buy our books directly from us at sliding scale rates? Support a small, independent publisher and pay less than Amazon's price at **www.Microcosm.Pub**.

CONTENTS

FOREWORD

As all mushroom fans know, eating little fun-guys, as I like to call them, can be a trying experience. As much as we love and appreciate them, none of us enjoy the sensation of chewing on dried out, fibrous fungi stalks. Our experiences learning to integrate small, measured quantities of shrooms into food and drink inspired us to collaborate in our kitchen on this definitive guide to cooking with shrooms.

We hope that it helps you experience your fun-guys in new, healthful, and meaningful ways. With that in mind, we have decided to make all the recipes as health conscious as possible—while still being delicious and a little indulgent from time to time. You'll find that everything here has no added sugars and is lactose-free; we have also included gluten-free substitutions throughout. Happy cooking, and best wishes as you embark on your journey with food and fungi!

We would like to include a quick word on safety and intentional psychedelic use. The ideal dose in all our recipes is usually one gram per serving or less, though this may vary. Keeping track of your dosages, particularly if making and consuming multiple recipes, is critical to ensuring you have a safe and enjoyable experience. Unintentionally consuming more than your intended dose can lead to an unexpectedly intense experience, or even a bad trip.

Individuals diagnosed with, or at risk for mental health conditions that may include elements of psychosis (detachment from consensus reality), Bipolar I disorder, and schizophrenia should abstain from using psychedelics, unless under the supervision of a licensed, experienced mental healthcare professional. Because these types of conditions have a genetic basis, individuals with a parent diagnosed with either condition should be particularly careful about their use of psychedelics.

Individuals who are prescribed psychiatric pharmaceuticals should also be mindful of their use of psychedelics. Commonly prescribed drugs, including SSRIs, SNRIs, and MAOIs, interact with psychedelics and can lead to serotonin syndrome. MAOIs are also present in some foods, such as yogurt, aged cheeses, and other fermented foods. St. John's Wort, a common nutritional supplement, is also an MAOI. Individuals who are prescribed benzodiazepines should keep in mind that those pharmaceuticals counteract psychedelics. If you choose to use, please respect your body, mind, and spirit by being mindful of the other chemical factors involved. TripSit's Guide to Drug Combinations is a helpful visual resource (tripsit.me), and The Vaults of Erowid (erowid.org/psychoactives/) contain extensive qualitative reports of drug experiences.

Harm Reduction and Safety

There should be a balance between these two primary layers of the psychedelic experience. If one of these is out of equilibrium, the other should compensate for this distortion. For example, if someone chooses to ingest a psychedelic in order to process trauma, their external environment should be curated by the traveler and the sitter (a trusted person who can stay with you during your trip) to serve as a safe container for the experience. If the setting is more unpredictable, such as a music festival, concert, or other gathering, the responsible psychonaut will be sure that their internal state is at equilibrium before choosing to ingest any substances.

These concepts lead to the foundation of psychedelic peer support. Organizations such as Kosmicare and Zendo Project collaborated on a beautiful book, entitled *The Manual of Psychedelic Support*, that was published by the Multidisciplinary Association for Psychedelic Studies (MAPS). The book details the philosophy of psychedelic support, and explains at length the four principles of psychedelic support:

1. Safe space. If someone is having a challenging experience, try to move them into a comfortable, warm, and calm environment. If possible, try to avoid noisy or crowded spaces. Ask what would make them most comfortable. Offer blankets and water.

2. Sitting, not guiding. Be a calm meditative presence of acceptance, compassion, and caring. Promote feelings of trust and security. Let the person's unfolding experience be the guide. Don't try to get ahead of the process. Explore distressing issues as they emerge, and recognize that simply being with the person can provide support.
3. Talk through, not down. Without distracting from the experience, help the person connect with what they are feeling. Invite the person to take the opportunity to explore what's happening and encourage them not to resist it.
4. Difficult is not bad. Challenging experiences can wind up being our most valuable, and may lead to learning and growth. Consider that it may be happening for an important reason. Suggest that they approach the fear and difficult aspects of their experience with curiosity and openness.

You can find more invaluable resources online at zendoproject.org. You can also download The Manual's full text for free at psychsitter.com.

Integrating Your Psychedelic Experience

Integrating a psychedelic experience is a crucial step in the journey of psychedelic use, especially when these substances are approached for their potential therapeutic benefits or for personal growth. Integration, in the context of psychedelics, refers to the process of assimilating the insights, emotions, and visions encountered during a psychedelic experience into one's daily life. It's about making sense of what was experienced during the altered state of consciousness and applying it in a way that promotes healing, personal development, and a greater understanding of oneself and one's place in the world.

The importance of integration cannot be overstated because the psychedelic experience can often be profound, overwhelming, and life-altering. Without proper integration, the insights gained can remain abstract, confusing, or even distressing, failing to produce lasting positive change. Integration helps individuals process their experiences, allowing them to extract meaningful lessons and insights that can lead to significant personal transformation. This process often involves discussing the experience with a therapist or guide, journaling, meditation, and other reflective practices that help translate the psychedelic journey into actionable steps for personal growth.

Moreover, integration is essential for grounding the individual after the often-intense emotional and psychological effects of psychedelics. It provides a safe space for individuals to unpack their experiences, confront any challenging or negative aspects they encountered, and begin healing any psychological wounds that were revealed. With integration, the individual can work through these challenges constructively, turning potential trauma into a catalyst for resilience and understanding.

Integration also supports the broader societal acceptance and understanding of psychedelics. By emphasizing the importance of thoughtful, responsible use and the work that comes after the experience, integration helps to dispel the misconceptions about psychedelics being merely recreational drugs. It highlights their potential as tools for profound personal and spiritual growth, encouraging a more respectful and mindful approach to their use. In doing so, integration not only benefits the individual but also contributes to a cultural shift towards recognizing the value of psychedelics in mental health, wellness, and personal development.

A Quick How-To for Cooking with Fun-Guys

Cooking with fun-guys, AKA Magic Mushrooms, is a wonderfully fun and engaging process. Sure, there are a ton of ways you can ingest our fungal friends, but taking the time to prepare a meal, with love and effort, engenders a greater connection between the psilocybin containing fellas and our souls. When I wrote this book, my purpose was to give people new and creative ideas for incorporating psilocybin into a weekly micro-dosing routine, but I understand that that may not be your cup of tea.

With that in mind, here are a few rules for cooking with Magic Mushrooms and increasing (or decreasing) the dosage.

Rule 1: High heat is a trip killer.

Whenever you're baking, stewing, or brewing these fellas, remember that our goal is to cook them low and slow. Don't exceed temperatures greater than 425 degrees for periods longer than 15 minutes. So, for example, if you are making our wonderful pumpkin pie and you'd like the edges nice and golden brown, bake it at 425 for 15 minutes, then lower the temperature to 350 degrees for the remainder.

Rule 2: When it's dry try 1:1.

Whenever you're cooking with dry ingredients and you want to increase or decrease your dosage but need to retain the proper dry-to-wet ratio, follow this rule. Add or subtract one-part dry ingredient, such as flour, for every gram of Magic Mushrooms you add or take away. This will help our baked goods maintain their consistency and not get too tough, dry, or wet. One quick note, if you are adding massively more psilocybin than the recipe calls for, you may need to adjust this to 1:1/2 ratio of dry to dry. i.e. add one gram of powdered mushrooms to a batter and take away half a gram of flour.

Dosage (Dried Psilocybin Mushrooms)	Experience Level	Expected Effects
Microdose (0.1g - 0.3g)	Sub-perceptual	May improve mood, creativity, and focus without noticeable psychedelic effects.
Low Dose (0.3g - 1g)	Mild	Mild euphoria, slight sensory enhancement, and increased emotional awareness without significant hallucinations.
Museum Dose (1g - 2.5g)	Moderate	Enhanced colors, visual patterns, emotional introspection, and philosophical thought. Altered perception of time and space.
High Dose (2.5g - 5g)	Strong	Intense visual and auditory hallucinations, profound insight or spiritual experiences, and a strong sense of connectivity. Possible loss of reality.
Heroic Dose (5g and above)	Very Strong	Extremely intense experience. Deeply introspective or mystical experiences. Not recommended for inexperienced users.

Rule 3: Everything in moderation.

Our recipes are designed with smaller doses, but they can be "leveled up" to increase the potency. If you're going to do this, then simply add the desired amount. However, please be safe and keep your dosage in mind, especially if you are making more than one recipe from the book (some are best in pairs).

Remember, this chart is a guideline, not a prescription. Individual experiences with psilocybin can vary significantly. Always prioritize safety, consent, and informed decision-making in any psychedelic experience.

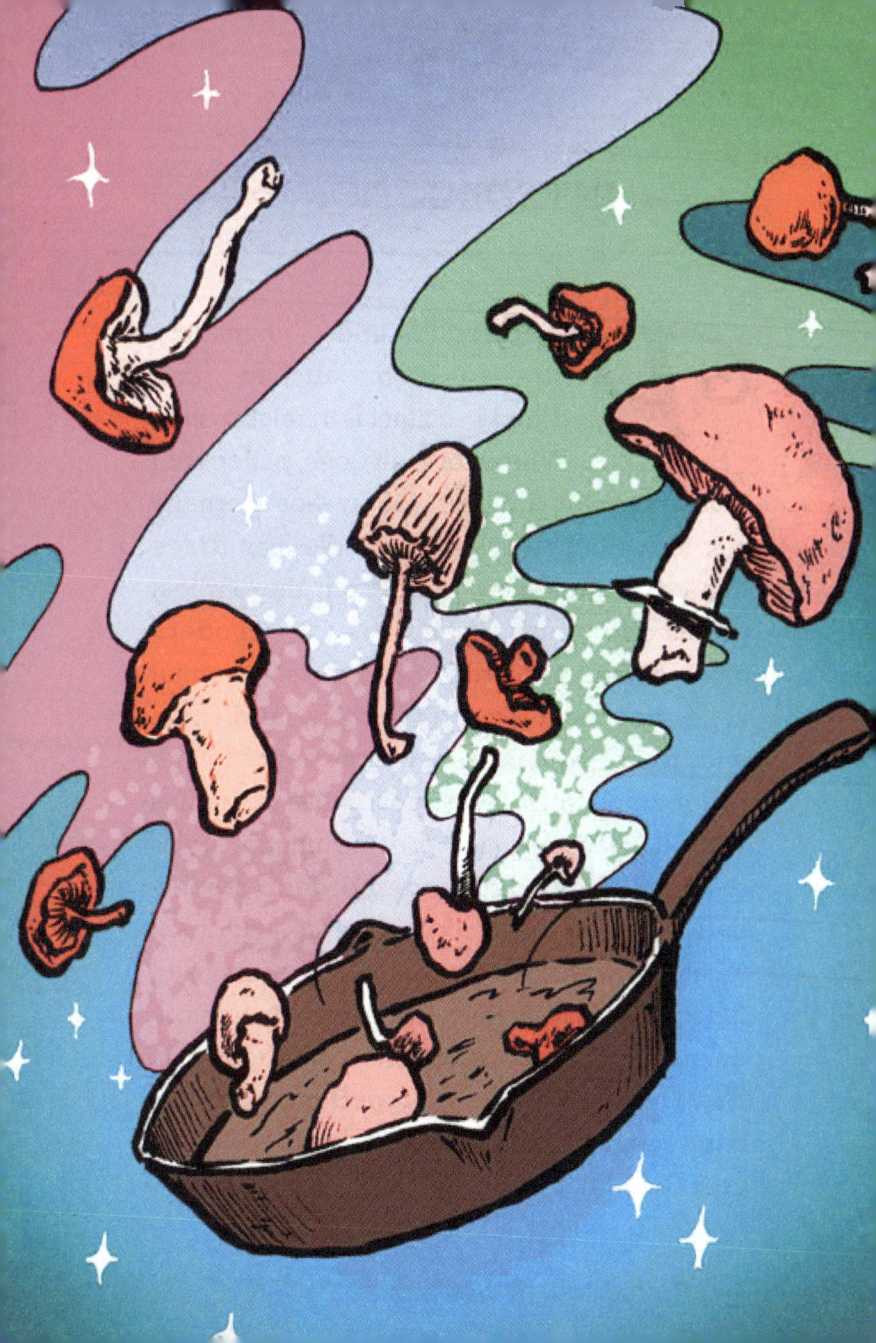

INTRODUCTION

Psilocybin and humanity have a rich, ancient, and deeply connected relationship. Wherever man goes, psilocybin containing mushrooms follow—or perhaps it's the other way around. We can trace this co-evolutionary bond from the earliest prehistoric cave paintings to modern studies that explore psilocybin's potential as a treatment for depression, addiction, and more. My personal experiences with psilocybin, during my post-military battles with depression and post-traumatic stress disorder (PTSD), engendered deep respect and a driving curiosity to explore and share what knowledge I can about this amazing fungal ally of humanity. This desire to explore an ancient relationship—how we found it, how we lost it, and most importantly, how we can regain it—were the driving factors in the creation of this book.

The main way I explore and use Magic Mushrooms is through food. I believe that by connecting psilocybin use with cooking, we deepen the spiritual and emotional aspect of using this potent psychedelic. This is backed up by history itself. For as long as we have had fire, man has consumed Magic Mushrooms in various forms, whether it be wines, teas, food, or just by themselves. It makes sense that we should take the act of feeding yourself, or your friends and family, something that for thousands of years was an act of love and consideration, and bind our use of psychedelics to the purely human ritual of cooking and sharing food. In fact, I have grown quite fond of adapting our daily microdosing routine into the creation of pies, main dishes, drinks, and more. I have selected a handful of these recipes to share, in the hope that it will inspire others to do the same.

A HUMAN HISTORY WITH PSILOCYBIN

CHAPTER ONE

The ancient use of psilocybin, the psychoactive compound found in over 200 species of mushrooms, is a subject that fascinates historians, archaeologists, and ethnobotanists alike. While direct evidence from prehistoric times is scarce due to the perishable nature of mushrooms, indirect evidence such as rock art suggests that humans have been interacting with psychoactive substances, possibly including psilocybin mushrooms, for thousands of years. One of the most compelling pieces of evidence is the rock paintings in the Tassili n'Ajjer plateau of Algeria, dating back to around 9000-7000 BCE, which depict figures with mushroom-like objects in their hands, leading some to speculate about the use of hallucinogenic mushrooms in prehistoric rituals.

In Mesoamerica, the historical record becomes clearer. The Aztecs referred to psilocybin mushrooms as *teonanácatl*, translating to "flesh of the gods," a name that underscores the sacred status these mushrooms held within their culture. Consumed during religious ceremonies, these mushrooms were believed to facilitate communication with deities, allowing shamans and laypeople alike to gain spiritual insight, divine the future, or seek healing. Spanish chroniclers, arriving in the 16th century, documented their use, albeit with a mix of fascination and horror, as they witnessed firsthand the profound effects these substances had on indigenous practices and beliefs.

The Mazatec people of Oaxaca, Mexico, provide a more contemporary glimpse into the ancient ritualistic use of psilocybin mushrooms. For the Mazatecs, these mushrooms are sacred, used in healing ceremonies that are deeply spiritual and therapeutic. The rituals are typically conducted by a *curandero* or *curandera* (a healer) who guides the participant through their experience, invoking Catholic saints and indigenous deities in a syncretic blend of pre-Hispanic and Christian traditions. This practice, which has been passed down through generations, underscores the continuity of psilocybin use from ancient times to the present day.

Greek Mysteries and their Psychedelic Origins

The question of ancient Greek or related cultures using psilocybin specifically is a matter of speculation and interpretation, as direct evidence is scarce. The ancient Greeks, renowned for their explorations of the mind, spirituality, and medicine, certainly used various psychoactive substances in their religious and healing practices, but the historical record does not explicitly mention psilocybin mushrooms.

One of the most intriguing connections between ancient Greek culture and the use of psychoactive substances is the Eleusinian Mysteries, secretive rituals held annually for over a thousand years in the town of Eleusis, near Athens. These rites were dedicated to

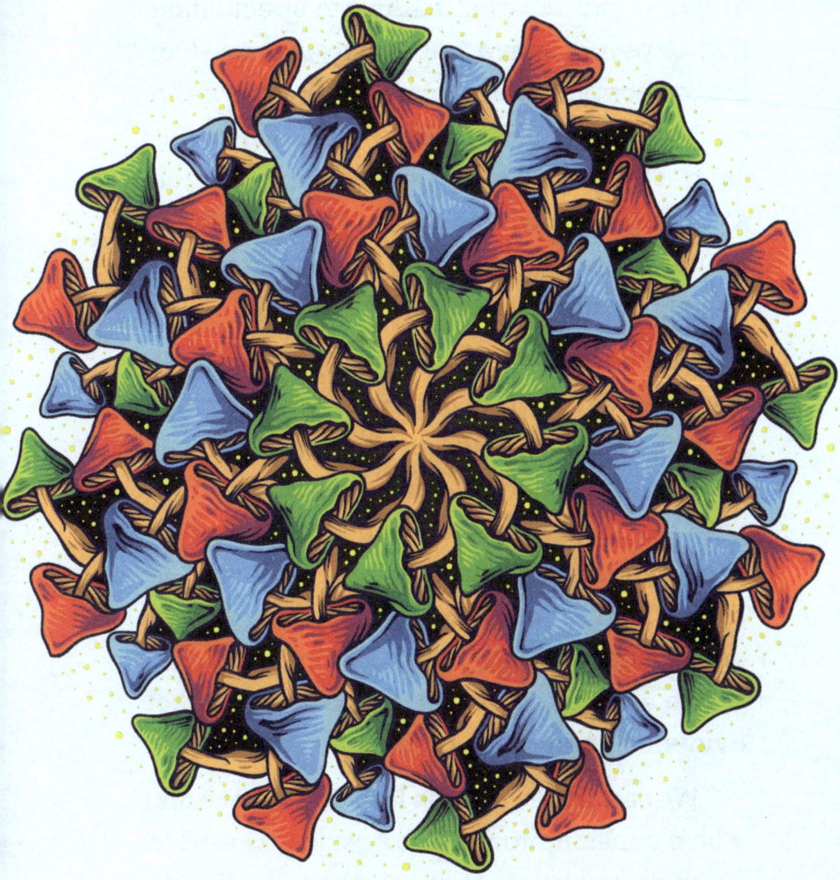

Demeter and Persephone and were central to Greek religious life. Participants reportedly experienced profound visions and a sense of dying and rebirth, leading to speculation that a psychoactive substance was part of the *kykeon*, the ceremonial drink consumed during the rituals. While some theories suggest the drink may have contained ergot, a fungus from which LSD is derived, there is no concrete evidence to suggest that psilocybin mushrooms were involved.

Another speculative link to psychoactive use in ancient Greek culture is the Oracle of Delphi, where priestesses, known as *Pythias*, would inhale natural gasses seeping from the earth before delivering prophecies. While this trance-like state was attributed to divine inspiration, some have theorized that psychoactive substances could have played a role. However, again, there is no direct evidence linking this practice to psilocybin.

We can also look to the Dacian Sons of Ares, who's consumption of Fly Agaric was said to be their source of strength and unnaturally strong martial gifts. This bright red and white-spotted mushroom has psychoactive properties, primarily due to compounds like muscimol and ibotenic acid. The Roman historian, Trajan, explicitly documents this mushroom consumption during berserker rites, which were reportedly observed during the Roman conquest of Dacia. Could you imagine being a Roman legionary staring over the brim of your scutum at a line of mad, wolf-skinned Dacian warriors? I can barely suppress my own shivers thinking about the sheer awe and fear this must have instilled, even in the steadfast Romans.

Fairies, Toadstools, and Heroes of Ancient Ireland

At the same moment in time, the Thracian's Irish cousins far to the north were creating a rich, oral tradition with stories about the Tuatha de Danann, Fomorians, and Fairies. These tales have long been thought by a variety of historians and archaeologists to contain many thinly veiled references to visions imparted by the use of psychoactive mushrooms, likely Liberty Cap and Fly Agaric. Take the legend of Fionn mac Cumhail, whose magical hazelnuts were likely Liberty

Cap mushrooms, which, when consumed, granted him foresight and knowledge, as well as the ability to see things which normal men could not.

There is also the tale of Máel Dúin from around the 8th century. Máel was the son of a petty Irish king who, during his journey to avenge his father's death, encountered an "Isle of Intoxicating fruits." Upon drinking a tea made from these fruits, he entered a trance-like state where he found himself unable to move, and was imparted with visions. Doesn't this sound a bit like our old friend *Amanita muscaria*, aka Fly Agaric, which is known to occasionally cause temporary paralysis in high doses?

We also have the tales of Saint Brendan and his findings of euphoric fruits growing near the base of certain trees. However, the main problem we have here is that the Celts, unlike the ancient Greeks, didn't write much down. What we do have comes from outsiders looking in, such as Saint Brendan and Saint Patrick; in their mission to convert the natives to Christianity they may have purposefully failed to write about ancient Irish psychedelics. Despite this lack of concrete knowledge, it is easy to make the connection between their oral traditions of fairies, strange gods, and morphing landscapes, with the effects we know are caused by ingesting psychoactive fungus.

Viking Berserkers, Fueled by Trippy Truffles?

A more well-known tale of our ancestors and their possible use of Magic Mushrooms can be found with the Vikings and their revered berserkers. These mighty warriors were dedicated to Odin, from the Norse pagan pantheon, and were known to go into battle nude, or wearing only a wolf skin. It has long been a popular theory that the Berserkers would partake in the eating of *Amanita muscaria* before battle, and that this is what gave them their fearsome strength, joy for battle, and near immunity to pain. Of course it is important to note that as a society who passed down stories primarily via an oral tradition, it is impossible to say whether or not this is true.

Yet there is an unquestionable mystery and draw to the idea that these renowned and feared warriors went into battle fueled by our little fungi friends. They are said to have been so intoxicated by battle lust, drink, and other substances, that they would bite their shields and even lash out at allies. They were also notoriously difficult to control in battle, and were best left to their own devices rather than put into formation. This theory is dubious at best; anecdotal reports from those who have tried Fly Agaric have shown it to be a rather peaceful experience that does not lend itself to the ferocious mental state someone would have to be in to achieve the feats attributed to berserkers.

Reindeers of Siberia

Another mushroom-friendly culture can be found in Siberia. Siberian shamanic practices, particularly among indigenous groups such as the Evenks and the Koryaks, have long been associated with the use of psychoactive substances to induce altered states of consciousness for spiritual and healing purposes. One of the most intriguing aspects of these practices involves the use of the *Amanita muscaria* mushroom, also known as the Fly Agaric. Shamans consumed these mushrooms to embark on spiritual journeys, communicate with the spirit world, and perform healing rituals. The psychoactive effects of *Amanita muscaria* include altered perception, euphoria, and in some cases, visual hallucinations, which were integral to the shaman's role as a mediator between the human and spiritual realms.

While this type of interaction with our fungal friends is seen throughout history, the people of this area developed a rather unique way of preparing them. Reindeer are known to seek out and consume *Amanita muscaria* mushrooms, attracted by their intoxicating effects. The psychoactive compounds pass through the reindeer's system and can be excreted in the urine with their psychoactive properties still intact, albeit in a less toxic form. Shamans discovered that by drinking the urine of these reindeer, they could safely experience the mushroom's effects, avoiding the more harmful compounds that can cause sickness. This practice allowed them to achieve the desired spiritual states with fewer physical side effects, facilitating their shamanic duties and spiritual journeys.

This symbiotic relationship between humans, animals, and psychoactive plants in Siberian shamanism highlights the complex understanding these cultures had of their natural environment and its potential to affect the human psyche and spirit. The use of *Amanita muscaria* and the subsequent consumption of reindeer urine containing its psychoactive chemicals is a testament to the ingenuity of indigenous practices in navigating the challenges and opportunities presented by their surroundings. These traditions, while seemingly exotic or even bizarre to outsiders, are deeply rooted in a holistic view of the world that sees humans, animals, and plants as interconnected beings, each playing a role in the spiritual and physical health of the community.

Modern Man, Our Relationship with Magic Mushrooms, and How We Lost It

Let's skip forward a few centuries to the mid 1950's. In the United States, Magic Mushrooms and their use were considered nothing more than folklore until 1957, when Life Magazine published an article written by the Vice President of J.P. Morgan, R. Gordon Wasson. Mr. Wasson had recently taken a trip to Mexico where he had the most wonderful and enlightening experience, with what he referred to as "divine mushrooms." During the course of his trip he reported such amazing sights as mountains, rivers, and great celestial bodies of water. In the article he wrote for Life, Mr. Wasson never once spoke negatively of the experience—in fact he extolled the virtues of Magic Mushrooms and even went so far as to suggest they could have therapeutic and medicinal uses. His article would skyrocket psilocybin mushrooms into the public eye, and even draw support from acclaimed Oxford professor Robert Graves.

It must also be said that Mr. Wasson would have never been able to partake in his journey, and thus write his article, without the help of one incredible and lesser known figure in the annals of psilocybin/human history.

This, of course, is Maria Sabina, the Mezo American shaman who would act as Wasson's spiritual and ritual guide during his trip to Mexico. Maria, a practicing shaman and medicine woman, descended from a long, traditional line of female shamans. She was also the first contemporary shaman to allow a Westerner to observe and participate in the *veladas*, or healing journeys administered by Mezo-American shamans using psilocybin. This practice was a way for the shamans, or *curanderos*, to actively communicate with their God through the use of potent Psilocybe mushrooms. Maria would facilitate Mr. Wasson's trip, and thus open up the modern U.S. relationship with psilocybin.

Opening this door would spell disaster for Maria. Following Wasson's article, the subsequent media attention thrust Maria into the spotlight, and she soon found herself besieged by Westerners seeking to partake in the very *veladas* she had shared with

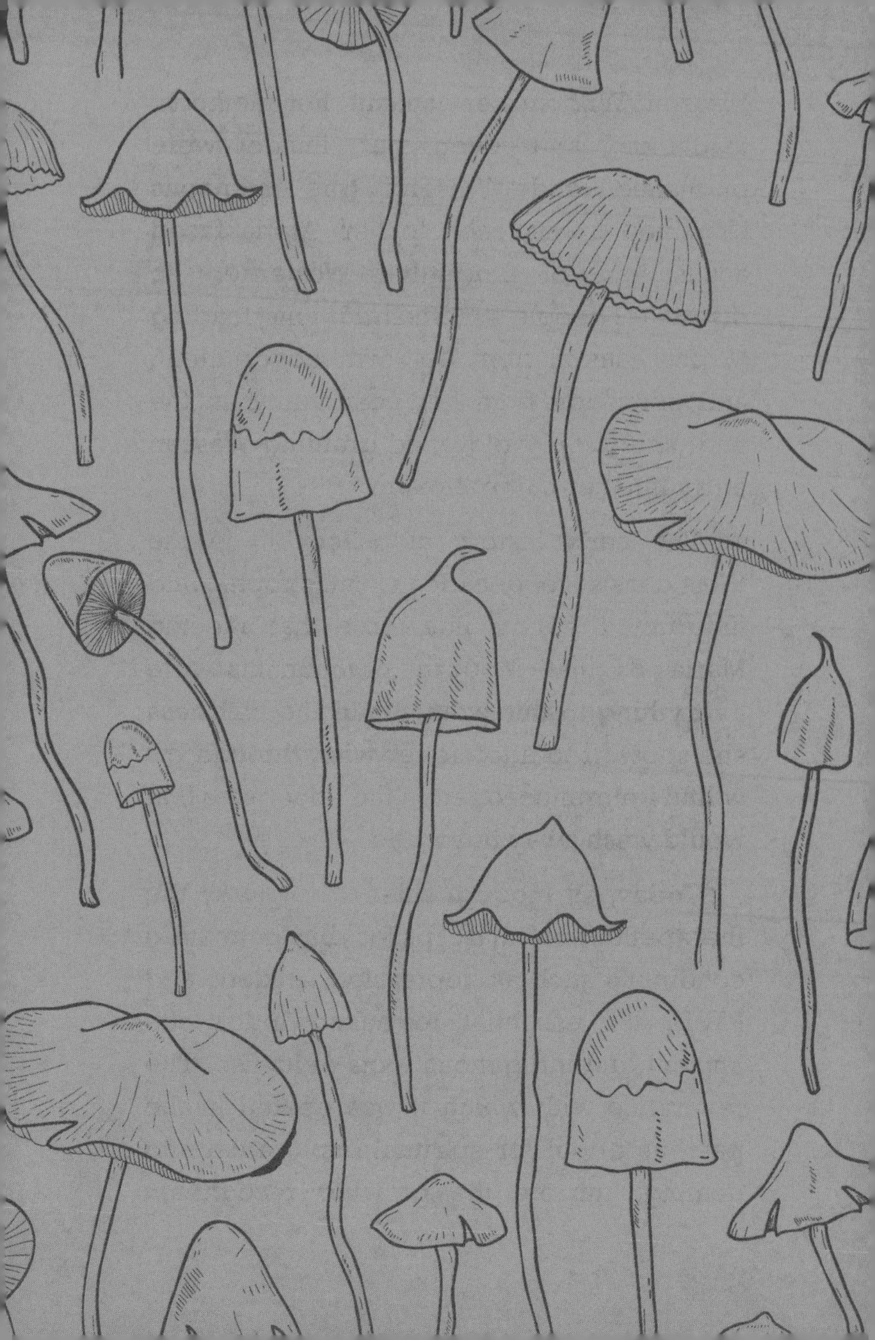

Wasson. Without her consent, her methods, teachings, and even her image were published, and Wasson's true intentions remained undisclosed to her. Maria faced accusations of permitting Westerners to distort her people's sacred traditions, leading to persecution from her own government, and alienation from her community. In the end, she deeply regretted granting Wasson entry into her cultural realm.

The early history of psilocybin in the West consists of decades of catastrophic and unfortunate events like those that affected Maria Sabina. Modern psychonauts owe everything to this woman and the kindness she showed to a foreigner who, through his willful ignorance, opened the floodgates that would wash away her world.

Today, as modern science explores the therapeutic potential of psilocybin for treating conditions such as depression, anxiety, and PTSD, it's essential to acknowledge the ancient and indigenous roots of its use. The reverence with which it was treated in the past, as a tool for spiritual exploration and healing, mirrors the growing recognition of its potential benefits. By understanding and respecting the historical and cultural contexts of psilocybin use, contemporary society can better appreciate the complex relationship humans have with this powerful psychoactive substance, bridging ancient wisdom with modern healing practices.

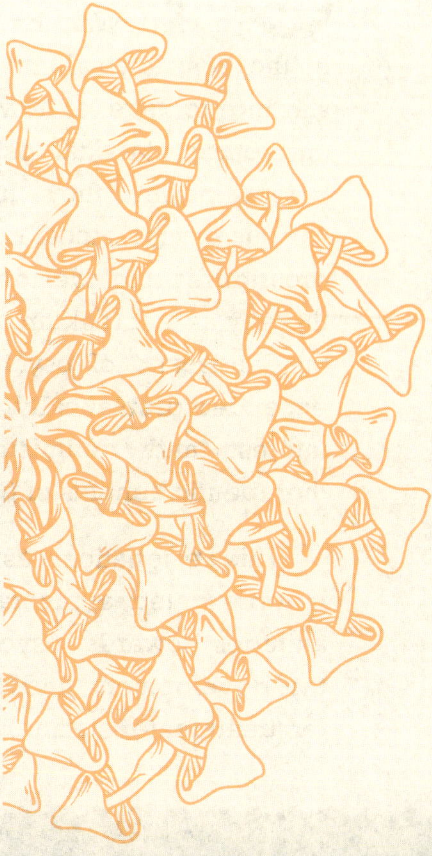

OUR RELATIONSHIP WITH PSILOCYBIN

CHAPTER TWO

After the debacle of psychedelic prohibition in the late 1960s, and the overall failure of the War on Drugs that began in the 70s, lawmakers and researchers are starting to take a new look at psilocybin and other classical psychedelics, and the potent power they have for combating various psychological issues. Since the FDA's groundbreaking designation of psilocybin therapy as a "breakthrough therapy" in 2018, the landscape of psychedelic research has expanded dramatically, reflecting a renewed interest and optimism in the potential therapeutic benefits of psilocybin.

This designation was not merely symbolic; it represented a pivotal shift in regulatory attitudes towards psychedelics, facilitating the development and review of psilocybin for treatment-resistant depression and other conditions. The impact of this decision has been profound, catalyzing a surge in clinical trials and research efforts aimed at exploring the full spectrum of psilocybin's therapeutic potential. Today, contemporary research is slowly being resurrected by scientists all over the world, from the brilliant minds at Johns Hopkins University and UCLA to the U.S. Department of Veterans Affairs.

The main focus of much of this research is in the field of end-of-life care and depression. Charles Grob, of UCLA, has conducted some brilliant work using psilocybin to ease the effects of depression and anxiety in patients suffering from advanced-stage cancer. His placebo-controlled study saw 12 patients given psilocybin in a double-blind study. The results were remarkable. The group given psilocybin, which was chosen over LSD due to its relatively short active period and ease of control, showed a significant drop in anxiety, fear, and depression, as well as a reduction in pain.

These effects carried on beyond the study, with patients reporting that their overall outlook was improved, and the reduction in their anxiety and depression continued for a notable period after the initial dose of psilocybin had been administered. Research and results of this magnitude are incredibly exciting; what more could we hope for from a drug that is widely considered safe (there is no known deadly dose of psilocybin, although I strongly condemn testing this out yourself) and non-addictive? If this style of work continues and the efficacy of psilocybin-based treatment becomes widely known, we could see ourselves at the forefront of a new and incredibly exciting revolution in the ways we treat severe anxiety and depression.

Now let's look at Johns Hopkins University, where a study into psilocybin-assisted psychotherapy is ongoing. This research, led by Roland Griffiths, and aimed at patients with early non-terminal cancer, found that psilocybin engendered positive improvement in mood, empathy, and behavior. These results were, for many of the patients, not just positive, but profoundly mystical and spiritual. These sessions were administered by knowledgeable and trained staff, and the patients were given eye masks and headphones to listen to music. The psilocybin reportedly gave participants a deep sense of sacredness, spiritualism, and an enduring sense of greater wellbeing and improved mental health. Griffiths reported that 80% of his patients disclosed that this was one of the most significant experiences of their lives, with the long-term effects being sustained for over a year.

Research into psilocybin's efficacy has broadened significantly in recent years, extending beyond the initial focus on depression to encompass a variety of mental health conditions that have historically been challenging to treat. Studies targeting PTSD (Post-Traumatic Stress Disorder) have begun to shed light on psilocybin's ability to alleviate the intense, often debilitating symptoms associated with traumatic experiences. Similarly, research into OCD (Obsessive-Compulsive Disorder) has explored how psilocybin therapy can potentially reduce the severity of compulsions and obsessions, offering hope to those for whom traditional treatments have fallen short. Additionally, the exploration of psilocybin as a treatment for eating disorders, including anorexia nervosa and binge eating disorder, is particularly promising, suggesting that psilocybin may help address the complex psychological components of these conditions.

Okay, so what have we learned so far? Psilocybin is proving to be an effective tool for the treatment of end-of-life distress, anxiety, and treatment-resistant depression. But what about some more everyday issues? Doctor Griffiths has also provided us with some interesting research into how psilocybin can be used to fight addiction.

Griffiths reports that a study conducted by his team, targeted at patients with a smoking addiction, showed a six month cessation of cigarettes after a single session dose of psilocybin. That is clearly a massive finding! What would our culture's long-term health outlook be if individuals suffering from addiction could check into a clinic and, after being administered a single, above-threshold dose of psilocybin, walk out of their doctor's office and leave behind a life of harmful drug or alcohol use? We spend around $170 billion dollars a year on cancer treatment for cigarette users (don't misunderstand this,

I am in no way passing judgment). What if, through the use of psilocybin and other classical psychedelics, we could reduce that to zero? It may seem implausible now, but as research continues and the public becomes more aware of psilocybin's powerful medical uses, we could one day live in a world where addiction is treated in a comfortable and caring environment, with caregivers administering this unbelievable psychedelic fungi.

The global recognition of psilocybin's potential is further evidenced by the establishment and expansion of dedicated research centers, such as the Centre for Psychedelic Research at Imperial College London. These institutions are at the forefront of psychedelic science, conducting rigorous studies that not only aim to understand the mechanisms by which psilocybin exerts its effects but also to develop protocols for its safe and effective therapeutic use. The work being done at these centers is multidisciplinary, involving psychologists, neuroscientists, and pharmacologists, among others, all collaborating to unlock the mysteries of psilocybin and translate their findings into clinical applications.

This burgeoning field of research represents a significant departure from the skepticism and legal barriers that once stifled psychedelic science. As studies continue to demonstrate the safety and efficacy of psilocybin for a growing list of conditions, the potential for psilocybin to revolutionize mental health treatment becomes increasingly apparent. With each new discovery, the promise of psilocybin as a versatile therapeutic agent becomes more tangible, heralding a new era in the treatment of mental health disorders and offering hope to millions of individuals worldwide.

We should also look at benefits outside of the medical aspect. Magic Mushrooms and their users report a greater sense of spirituality and worldly connectedness than non-users. Griffiths, again, shows that his patients, when asked about their post-psilocybin experience, felt as if they had a new understanding of the world on a more mystical level. This lines up with what we know of cultures with a long history of psilocybin use.

In a world plagued by climate change, sectarian violence, deforestation, and unfettered capitalism, we could really use a greater sense of connection with the earth and our fellow man. Perhaps if research is allowed to expand further, we could see psilocybin being used to treat more than just mental health issues and addiction, but societal ails like narcissism, greed, or even apathy

For a more indepth review of the state of medical research into psychedelics, take a look at *Acid Test* by Branden Schroder, and *Psychology of the Future* by Stan Grof. MAPS, the Beckley Foundation, and the Usona Institute, are also excellent sources for reference, as the subject material is too broad to be covered in depth in the few short pages available in this cookbook.

MICRODOSING

CHAPTER THREE

Microdosing is the practice of using and consuming psilocybin, and other psychedelics, in a sub-threshold or sub-perceptual dose (this means that the dose should be low enough that you feel little to no psychedelic effects). This process is typically used to increase creativity, energy, focus, and improve social awareness and empathy. It is thought that microdosing psilocybin works similarly to taking Selective Serotonin Reuptake Inhibitors, aka SSRIs, with one key difference. Where SSRIs stimulate increased serotonin output, psilocybin skips this step and directly mimics serotonin. The chemical structure of psilocybin, when converted into psilocin, so closely resembles our bodies naturally occurring serotonin, that uptake is rapid.

Psilocybin also has another key difference from SSRIs, an apparent lack of long-term side effects (this does not mean that there are none, just that there are currently no known long-term side effects from microdosing). SSRIs can cause users to experience side effects ranging from withdrawal, sexual dysfunction, weight gain, emotional numbness, and the development of suicidal thoughts and tendencies.

Another area of interest is the potential for microdosing to enhance creativity and problem-solving skills. Creatives and professionals in high-pressure industries have reported that microdosing helps them think more laterally, overcome creative blocks, and approach problems from novel perspectives. This is believed to be linked to psychedelics' ability to dampen the activity of the brain's default mode network (DMN), a network associated with self-referential thoughts and the ego. By reducing the dominance of the DMN, psychedelics could facilitate a more expansive state of mind, where ideas flow more freely and new connections are more easily made.

Despite these promising reports, the science of microdosing is still in its infancy, and there are significant controversies and challenges in the field. One major issue is the lack of large-scale, placebo-controlled studies, which are the gold standard in medical research. Much of the evidence for microdosing's benefits comes from self-reported data, which can be biased and unreliable. The placebo effect, particularly strong in studies involving psychoactive substances, could account for many of the positive outcomes reported by microdosers. Researchers are beginning to design more rigorous studies to overcome these limitations, but the results are still forthcoming.

There are also potential risks and side effects associated with microdosing. While psychedelics are generally considered safe and non-addictive, especially in low doses, there is concern about the long-term effects of regular microdosing. Some users report increased anxiety, physiological discomfort, or blurring of emotions over time. Furthermore, the legal status of psychedelics as Schedule I substances in many countries, including the United States, complicates research efforts and makes it difficult for individuals to safely and legally access these substances for microdosing.

What Else Does Our Little Fungal Friend Do?

Psilocybin ingestion leads to a few important effects that are thought to occur in the hippocampus. The first is the increased production of brain-derived neurotrophic factor (BDNF). BDNF is a supposed miracle chemical for your brain, as it stimulates the growth of new connections as well as the repair of old damaged connections.

It is also thought to be responsible for a psilocybin user's entrance into a more open and child-like state of mind. Do not confuse child-like with naive or simple, instead the increased production of BDNF allows your mind to become more open to new experiences and to more easily connect the dots when learning a new skill. This is similar to the way children's minds are more easily able to retain new information.

Children's brains are thought to be more adaptable than adults' due to the high levels of neuroplasticity during early development, which allows for easier formation and reorganization of neural connections in response to learning and experience. This heightened plasticity facilitates rapid learning and adaptation in childhood, a capacity that generally decreases with age. Psychedelics, like psilocybin may improve neuroplasticity in the adult brain, which in turn, may allow us to think in new ways, develop new neural pathways and approach problems with novel solutions.

The next important possible effect of microdosing is the uptick in production of glutamate; this is the neurotransmitter responsible for critical functions such as cognition, information retention, learning, and memory. It is thought that this increase in glutamate powers a microdoser's ability to quickly grasp and retain new information. It is also known to be responsible for increased interest in mundane tasks—which explains why the boys on Wall Street are happily consuming capsules packed with brain-enhancing psilocybin.

As discussed earlier, another aspect of the way our brain changes while microdosing is the suppression of the Default Mode Network. The Default Mode Network is the part of our brain that is responsible for things like day-dreaming, self-reflection, self-pity, and thinking about things that have happened in our past. While these of course are important functions, this part of the brain is often overworked, and some studies are linking an overactive Default Mode Network with depression and anxiety. This could explain why individuals who consistently use Magic Mushrooms report lower instances of depression and anxiety.

So What Exactly Is a Microdose?

Microdosing involves taking roughly a tenth of the dose that you would typically need to trip, so around 0.3 to 0.4 grams, if we assume that most people will achieve a trip level dose at around 3.5 grams. In my experience, anything over 0.5 grams makes you either a little too high to get anything done, or breaks into the sub-visual range of tripping and things will start getting a little weird.

I.e., you will either be oddly joyful, or wax philosophical for no apparent reason, which can make those boardroom meetings with your boss a bit awkward.

With that in mind, let's stick to the 0.3 grams range, which is currently all the rage in places like Silicon Valley and Wall Street, or the humble halls of college campuses across the country. This lower dose will provide the benefits of psilocybin consumption we are looking for, while avoiding issues like increased psilocybin tolerance, lack of focus, or just being a little too high to operate normally in your daily routine. You will of course also not be tripping—which I have been told can put a damper on your workday schedule.

When it comes to the kind of routine to follow for microdosing there are a few schools of thought. Some microdosers recommend taking them everyday, alternating days, or dosing on a one-day-on, two-day-off schedule. However, in this book, dosing everyday is not recommended for a variety of reasons. The first is the simple fact that psilocybin tolerance builds very quickly; if someone is dosing everyday, then within just two or three days they will see a significant drop in psilocybin's desirable effects. Heart-health is another reason not to dose everyday. Psychedelics, and psilocybin in particular, have been shown to cause ventricular hardening with extended daily use, which puts you at an increased risk for heart disease.

Now, let's talk about the first recommended dosing schedule covered here. This is a two week cycle with alternating one-day-on, one-day-off. For beginners, scaling your doses is highly recommended. The first time someone is microdosing, they should aim for a dose of 0.1 grams. Take one or two days off from work, school, or other responsibilities, and record how you feel. From there, you can scale as needed—up to that 0.3 gram sweet spot. The schedule should look something like on the following page:

Day 1 Dose 0.1 Grams	Off day	Day 2 Dose 0.2 Grams	Off day	Day 3 Dose 0.3 Gram	Off day	Off day
Day 4 Dose 0.3 Grams	Off day	Day 5 Dose 0.3 Grams	Off day	Day 6 Dose 0.3 Grams	Off day	Off day
			No Dose Week			

The addition of an entire week off from microdosing allows the body to reset and prepare for the following week. The next dose after taking that time off is much more potent and will really get those creative juices flowing. The no-dose week also allows your body to reset and should help prevent any long-term effects of dosing too regularly.

Another common dosing schedule is an off set one-day-on, two-day-off schedule. Some psychonauts find this schedule allows them to be more flexible and increases the punch of the microdose. For myself, I have found that there is not much difference between the perceived effects of an every-other-day schedule vs. the one-on, two-off schedule.

Day 1 Dose 0.1 Grams	Off day	Off day	Day 2 Dose 0.2 Grams	Off day	Off day	Day 3 Dose 0.3 Gram
Day 4 Dose 0.3 Grams	Off day	Off day	Day 5 Dose 0.3 Grams	Off day	Off day	Day 6 Dose 0.3 Grams
			No Dose Week			

Using the above schedule or the previous one is completely up to you. I would recommend that you experiment with them and even make up your own regiment. Microdosing, like tripping, is a very personal and deeply spiritual experience that should be tailored to fit your individual needs, goals, and lifestyle. Psilocybin is a powerful tool that should be used with purpose and intent. I hope this guide and the tables help you to learn, grow, and most of all, be safe when interacting with our magical fungi friends.

FUN-GUYS

CHAPTER FOUR

This section has been composed by our illustrator, Snowflake, who worked closely with the Erowid Foundation to ensure the illustrations in the section are not just beautiful, but also as scientifically accurate as possible.

There are well over 200 known species of psychoactive mushrooms across the planet, with many subspecies and a great many that are believed to be undiscovered as of yet. Some of these are common, some very rare. Some are easily found, some hide away in secretive places like mountainous cloud forests. Some are mild, some potent, while others are indeed toxic.

In this chapter you will see a few North American favorites, along with several others. These images are only meant as a visual reference guide for what you might happen across outside; this reference in no way provides instructions on how to cultivate them. The entries here are not intended for scientific education, but are well researched and intended to give you standard information in an easy-to-use reference.

Fungi will grow despite any laws against them; they are a defiant little bunch, and so having a way to identify what you may find in the wild will help you to be safer in your wanderings.

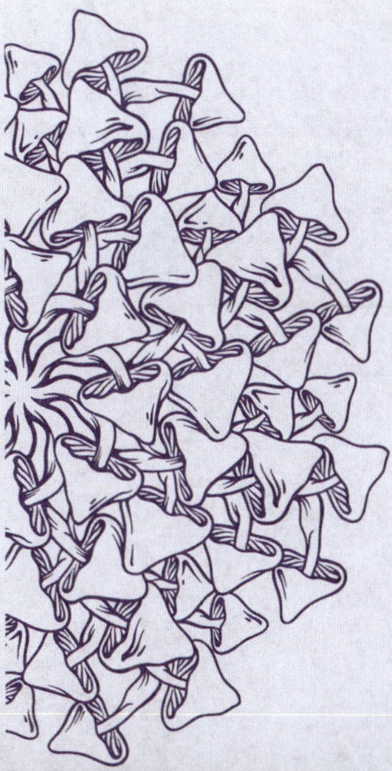

Psilocybe azurescens

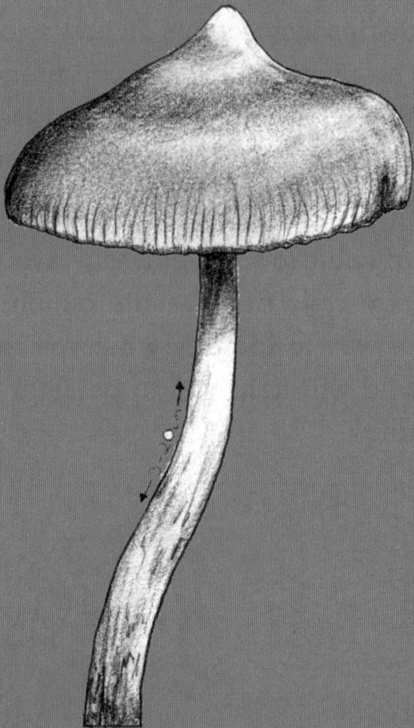

Also known as Flying Saucers, Copper Tops

Features

- This species thrives in unusually cold winter weather on the coastline
- This variety prefers dune grasses and beached wood

- They have the strongest concentration of all three psychedelic alkaloids ever discovered
- Grows typically in clusters
- Prominent nipple or *umbo*
- Caps grow 1.5-4 inches (3-10 cm) across
- These can be 4-8 inches (3-20 cm) tall, and the stem can get quite thick
- They are so potent, they bruise without effort

Range

- Limited range from coastal mid-Oregon to coastal mid-Washington
- Feral growths have been found in Germany
- Cultivable indoors

Colors

- Chestnut to caramel in gradient, drying to a straw color
- The cap bruises blue
- Has white gills and a white to brown fluffy base

Psilocybe baeocystis

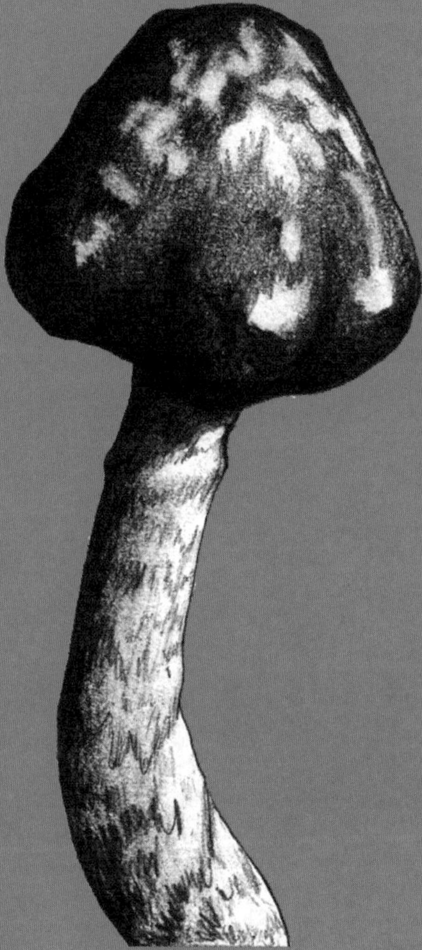

Also known as Bottle Caps, Knobby Tops, Blue Bells, Olive Caps

Features

- "Baeocystis" translates to "small bladder"
- Grows solitarily or in small clusters
- Bruises an intense blue easily, even from rain
- Potency is markedly greater when fresh, dropping by up to half when dry
- Caps are highly glossy when moist and grow anywhere from 1.5-2.5 inches (1.5-5.5 cm) across
- Stems grow 2-3 inches (5-7 cm) in length

Range

- Pacific Northwest
- Maine
- Can be cultivated at home

Colors

- Dark olive, brown, or greenish-brown
- Steel blue when wet
- Dries to a copper center with a white edge
- The gills are gray to cinnamon
- Stems are white to brownish

Psilocybe caerulipes

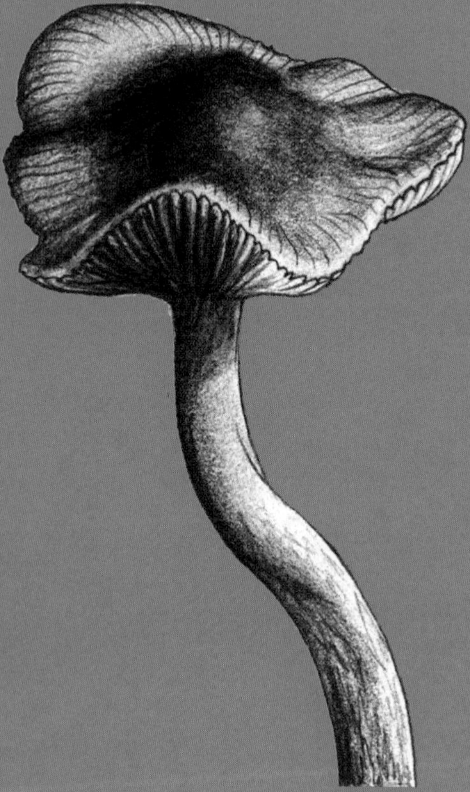

Also known as Bluefoots

Features

- These are often mistaken for the larger *P. ovoideocystidiata*

- They are very rare, having a wide and infrequent distribution
- These are solitary or in small clumps
- While there are cultivation methods, they are more difficult to grow and much stronger when fresh
- The caps begin small and concave, but open to a convex, often wobbly shape
- Caps are 0.5-1.5 inches (1-3.5 cm) across
- Stems grow to about 1.25-2.25 inches (3-6 cm) long

Range

- Most common in the Appalachian Range
- Can be found as far south as Mexico, in cloud forests

Colors

- The cap has a cinnamon to dingy brown gradient with a darker center
- The gills are rusty with pale edges
- Stems are brownish yellow to brown

Psilocybe cyanescens

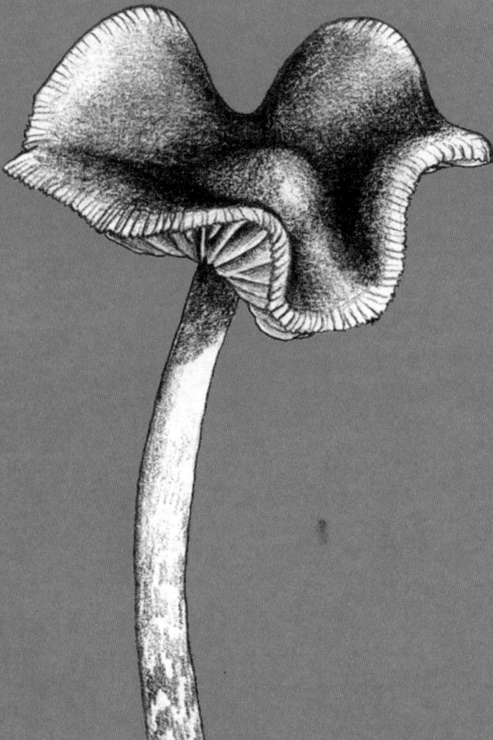

Also known as Wavy Caps, Potent psilocybe

Features

- This species prefers an unusually cool 50-65°F
- They can occur solo, but are most often found in large troops or even "fairy rings." Once instance in England reached 100,000 fruits in a single troop!

- Known for their potency
- There are several convincing toxic lookalikes, often growing nearby. Use caution!
- The iconic wonky caps are usually 1-2 inches (2-5 cm) when fully grown
- They grow from 1.5-3 inches (3.6 cm) tall
- At a young age, the cap is convex, with the waves showing in maturity

Range

- Found globally, most commonly in the Pacific Northwest
- These have cropped up all over the world due to distribution in mulch
- Can be cultivated indoors

Colors

- The caps are a gradient from a sienna center to a brownish-yellow edge
- Dries to much paler tones
- Cinnamon to dark-brown gills
- The stem is a smooth to silky white with blue bruising

Psilocybe mexicana

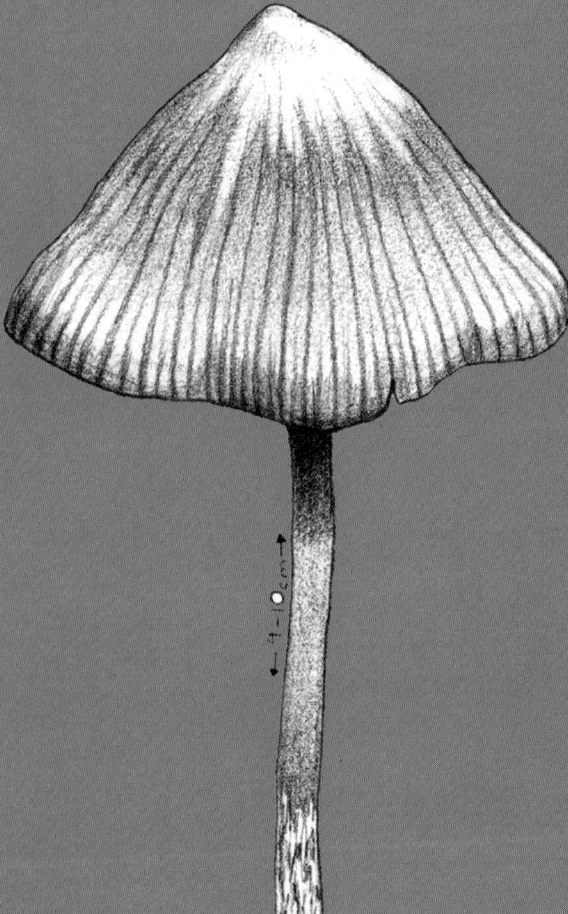

Also known as Teonanacatl (Aztec, meaning "God's flesh"), Chamaquillo, Little Bird

Features

- Grows either solo or in troops, prominently in high altitudes
- They have a notably small size
- Has thousands of years of recorded use
- This species is very common in appearance to *many* wild mushroom varieties, including poisonous species
- This species produces what are called "magic truffles" or *sclerotia*, a persistent, resting spore (see page 78)
- Caps grow from convex to concave, staying 1-2 inches (2-5 cm) in diameter
- Typically, the grow 2-4 inches (4-10 cm) in length

Range

- Mexico, Costa Rica, and Guatemala
- Has been found in the swamps of Florida, but this is extremely rare
- This species can be cultivated indoors

*Dr. Albert Hofmann first isolated psilocybin and psilocin with *p. Mexicana*

Psilocybe ovoideocystidiata

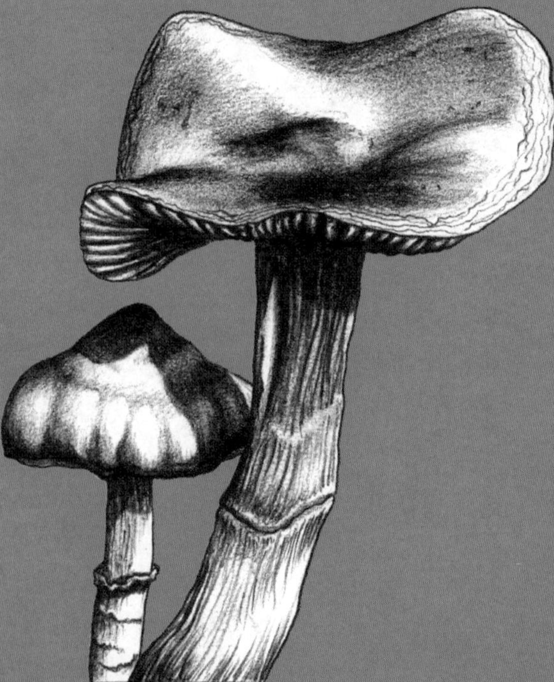

Also known as Ovoids, Bluefoots

Features

- The difference between growth stages are so dramatic, one image wouldn't be enough
- These grow in clusters. . . huge ones!
- They fruit every season except winter

- Most psilocybe species don't have a membranous ring, or *annulus*. Ovoids wear theirs halfway down their stems.
- There is no standard cultivation method
- Caps grow to be about 1.5-2 inches (3-5 cm) in diameter
- Stems can grow to up to 4 inches (9 cm)

Range

- Continental United States, Germany, and Switzerland

Colors

- In early stages, they are pearly cream to yellow/orange brown
- When mature, they are a mix of yellow, blue, and brown
- The caps exhibit dramatic blue and green bruising
- The gills range from rusty and white, to lavender and dark purple

Psilocybe pelliculosa

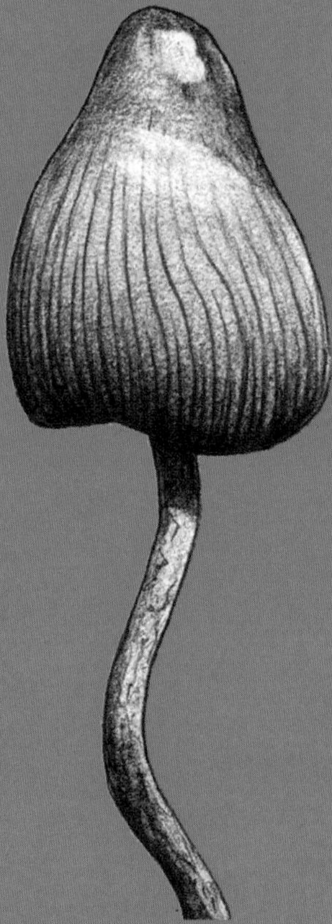

Also known as Conifer Psilocybe

Features

- Unlike most of the psilocybe fungi, this species barely bruises, it at all

- Grows in clusters and troops, and is harder to find
- Often found at elevations of 1000-2000 feet in clear-cuts where timber has been left
- They tend to grow on 3-10 year decaying conifer (evergreen) trees
- Caps stay convex throughout the fruiting process, growing to be about .25-1.5 inches (.5-3 cm)
- Stems are around 2.5-3 inches (6-8 cm)
- These prefer wet October through December
- No known indoor cultivation method

Range

- Northern Pacific Coast from Oregon through Alaska
- There is some feral growth in Finland

Colors

- Translucent chestnut brown when wet, drying to a range of yellows
- Gills are a cinnamon brown
- The stem is white to grayish, browning near the base

Psilocybe semilanceata

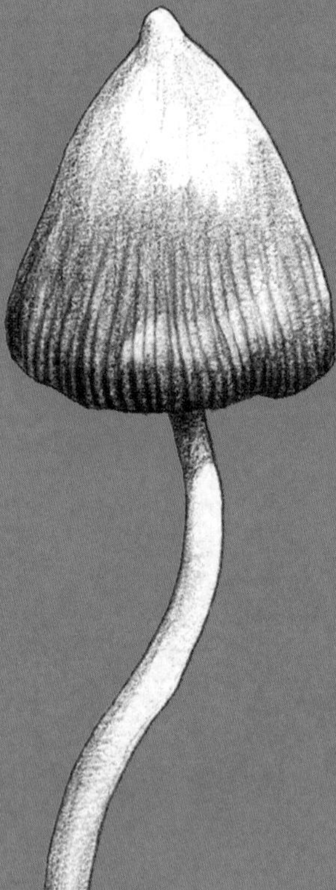

Also known as Liberty Caps, Magic Mushrooms

Features

- Cone-shaped cap with a prominent center nipple, or *umbo*
- Purple-brown spores

- These have a notably smaller stature, growing in troops or solo
- Typically, these grow in meadows used by sheep and cattle. However, unlike other species, they do not grow out of dung, but instead from decaying grass roots
- This species has *many* lookalikes, including poisonous varieties
- The caps typically do not grow beyond 1 inch (0.5-2.5 cm) across
- These grow to 2-4 inches (3-10 cm) tall

Range

- North American and Europe
- These have also been found in Peru, India, Australia, New Zealand, and even at altitudes of 4000m in Italy
- Can be cultivated indoors

Colors

- A dark chestnut brown when wet, drying to a light tan/yellow
- The gills are a purplish brown
- Off-white/tan stem

Conocybe velutipes

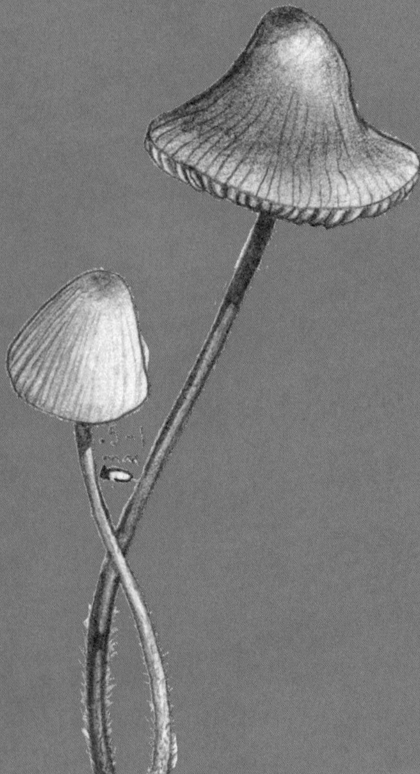

Also known as Okrakuupika (Finnish), Dunce Cap

Features

- This tiny, basic species looks nearly identical to a species that shares the toxin of the "death cap" mushroom, so beware

- Just like dozens of other species of common looking tiny brown fungi, this species is known as an "LBM," or Little Brown Mushroom
- Quite curiously, the spores if this species are elliptical
- Only one of five Conocybe species to be psychoactive
- These are usually found scattered in grass and woodlands
- These babies often have a dusting of mycelium fuzz on their fragile stems
- Caps are about 0.5 inches (1.2 cm)
- Stems grow to be about 1.5-2.5 inches (4-6 cm) tall

Range

- Concentrated in Illinois, the UK, and Sweden
- Found across North America and Europe

Colors

- Dull brown to yellowish-tan caps with a slightly darkened tip
- The gills match the cap, but then fade to a cinnamon color
- Stems are brown, frail, with a dainty mycelium dusting

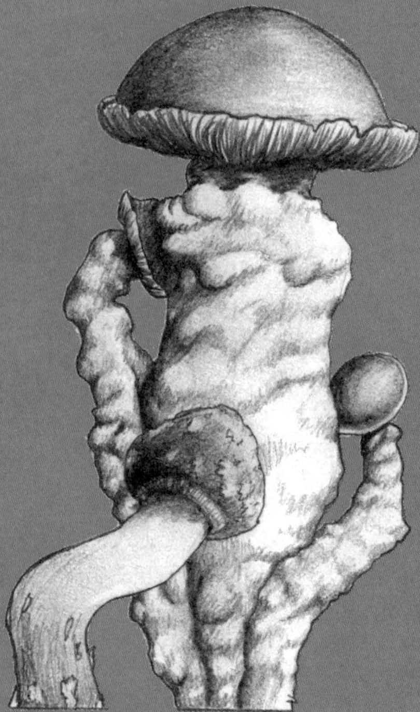

Also known as Cubes, Gold Tops, Penis Envy (strain specific)

Features

- *P. cubensis* has a fabulous variety of shapes, sizes, and colors. All of which depend on age, growth method, and strain or subspecies.

- These grow in clusters
- Shrink to up to a tenth of their original size when dried

Range

- Grows widely across Asia, North and South America, Oceania, and Africa
- Can be cultivated indoors

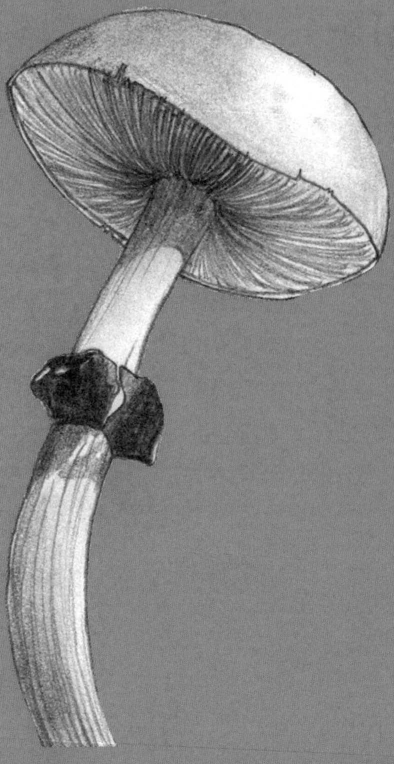

Sclerotia

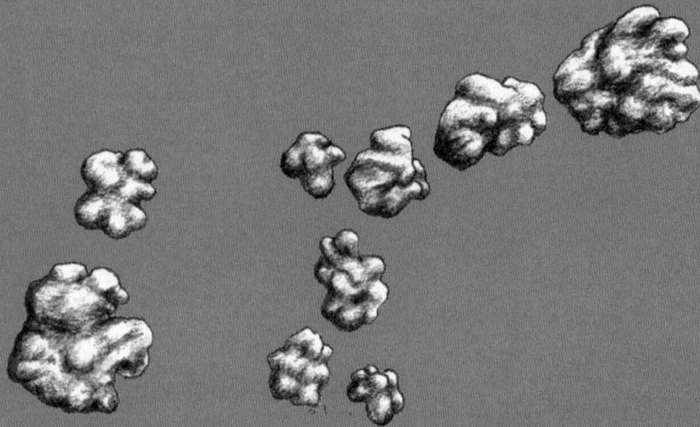

These are known to most as "magic truffles." However, these are not in fact a truffle species, but rather a different part of the above-ground mushroom we already know. They are a resting form of a variety of fungi that stay underground and persist through drought, frost, and even wildfires until conditions are right for the fungus to fruit.

Species

- Psilocybe tampanensis
- Psilocybe mexicana

Common Names

- Philosopher's Stones
- Tripknollen (Dutch)

- Space Truffles
- Magic Truffles

Features

- While not mushrooms, these do contain the active alkaloids that induce psychoactivity
- They come in a variety of browns and often have a "nutty" taste

The Helpful Guide to Outdoor Leavemalones

This guide is here to help you and your friends stay safe, and to be able to see right away what some of the most toxic varieties look like so you can steer clear of them. It is important to note that several of these resemble some of the edible varieties. For goodness sake, always be careful when handling any fungus you discover!

Many thanks to Fire and Earth Erowid for their insight and assistance in researching and preparing these illustrations. For more information on fungus research, please see the resources guide at the back of this book for some scientific sources to learn even more about Magic Mushrooms.

Deadly Webcaps

Cortinarius rubellus

Europe, North America

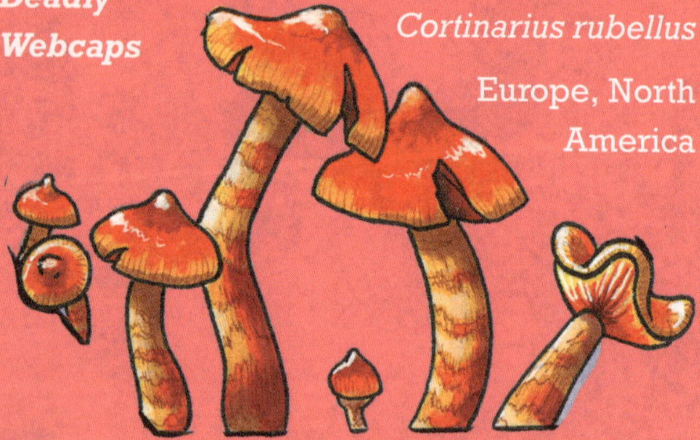

Death Cap

Amanita phalloides

Europe

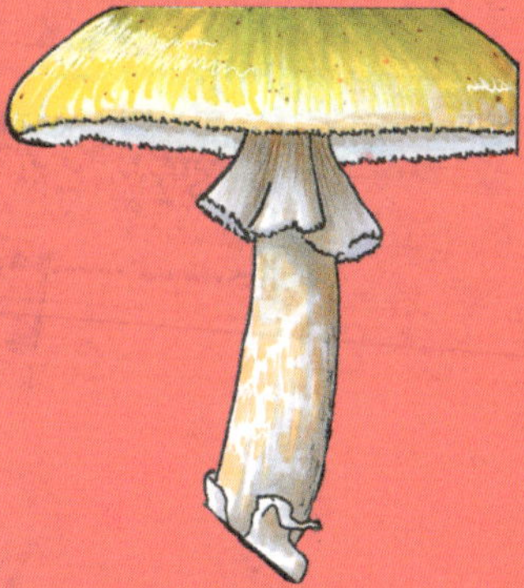

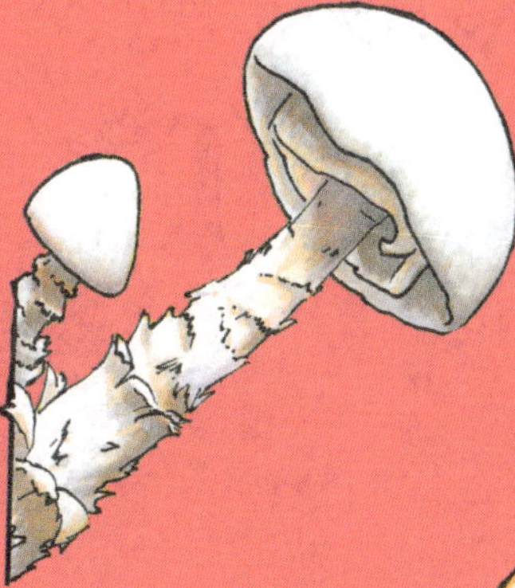

Destroying Angels

Amanita bisporigera

North America

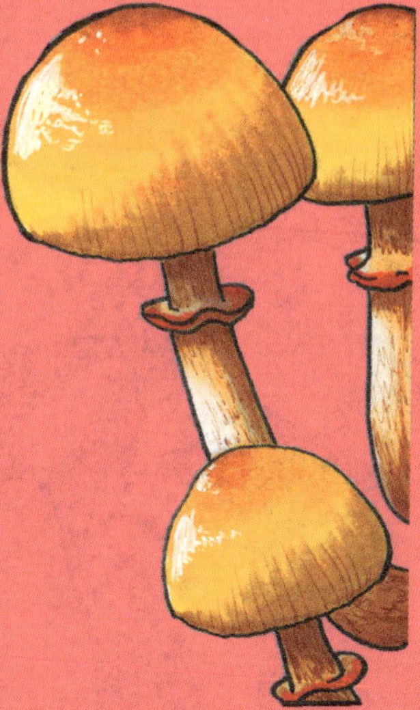

Deadly Galerina, or Funeral Bells

Galerina marginata

Global

Fly Agaric/Fly Amanita, Toadstool

Amanita Muscaria

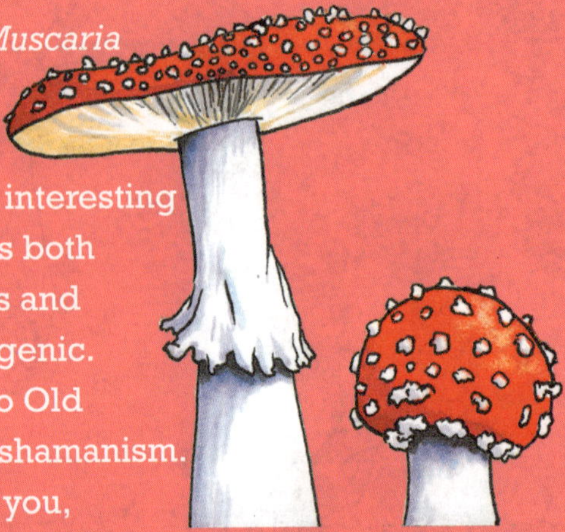

This is an interesting one as it is both poisonous and hallucinogenic. It is tied to Old Eurasian shamanism. I implore you, practice caution.

Global

Deadly Dapperling

Lepiota brunneoincarnata

Europe, Asia

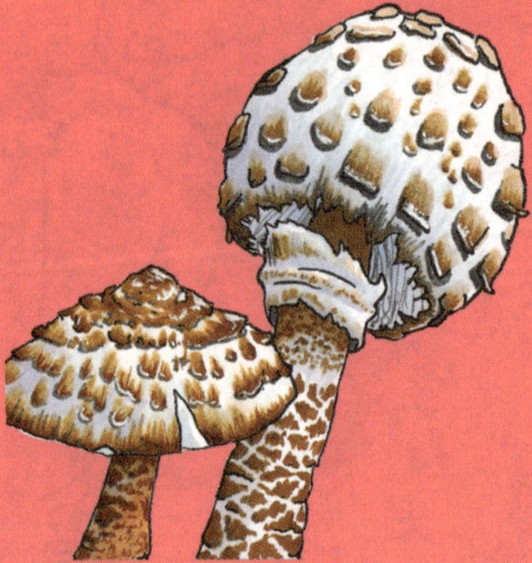

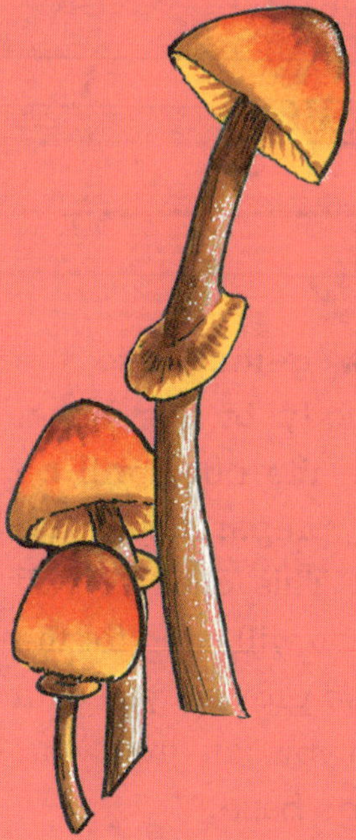

Common Lawn Mushroom

Conocybe filaris

These are deadly poisonous from amatoxins, are extremely common, and are easily mistaken for Psilocybe. Be Careful!

Europe, North America

Fire Flame Kinoko

Podostroma cornu-damae

Asia

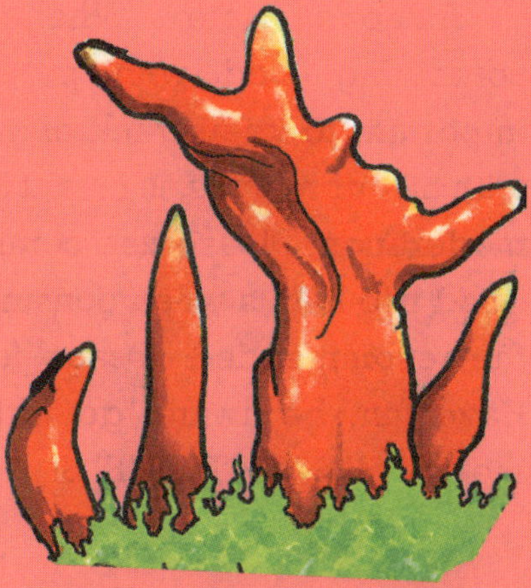

THE BASIC NECESSITIES

CHAPTER FIVE

We are now getting into the primary body of this book. From here, the book will be covering preparation and cooking with psilocybin. This chapter will cover the basics of what you will need for the recipes to come. It will also provide you with the foundation from which you can grow your experience and knowledge base.

Author's Note: Whenever you are combining food with psychedelics it is important to keep track of your dose. This, with all our recipes, is meant to be enjoyed in moderation. Please use common sense and good trip habits when consuming more than the recommended dosage for each recipe. Have fun, be aware, go with purpose and most of all SAFE TRAVELS!

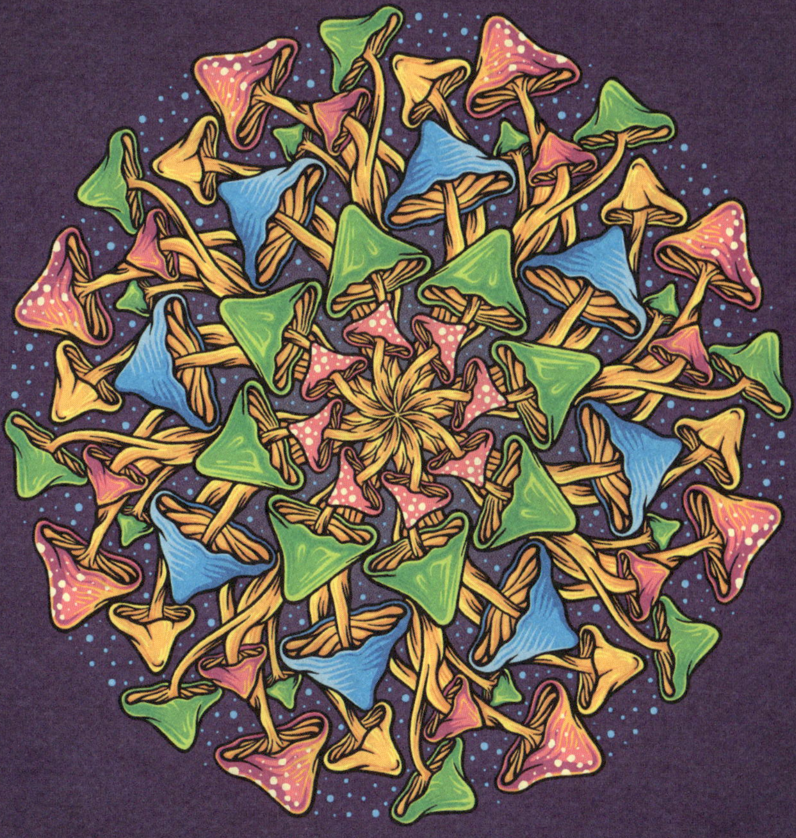

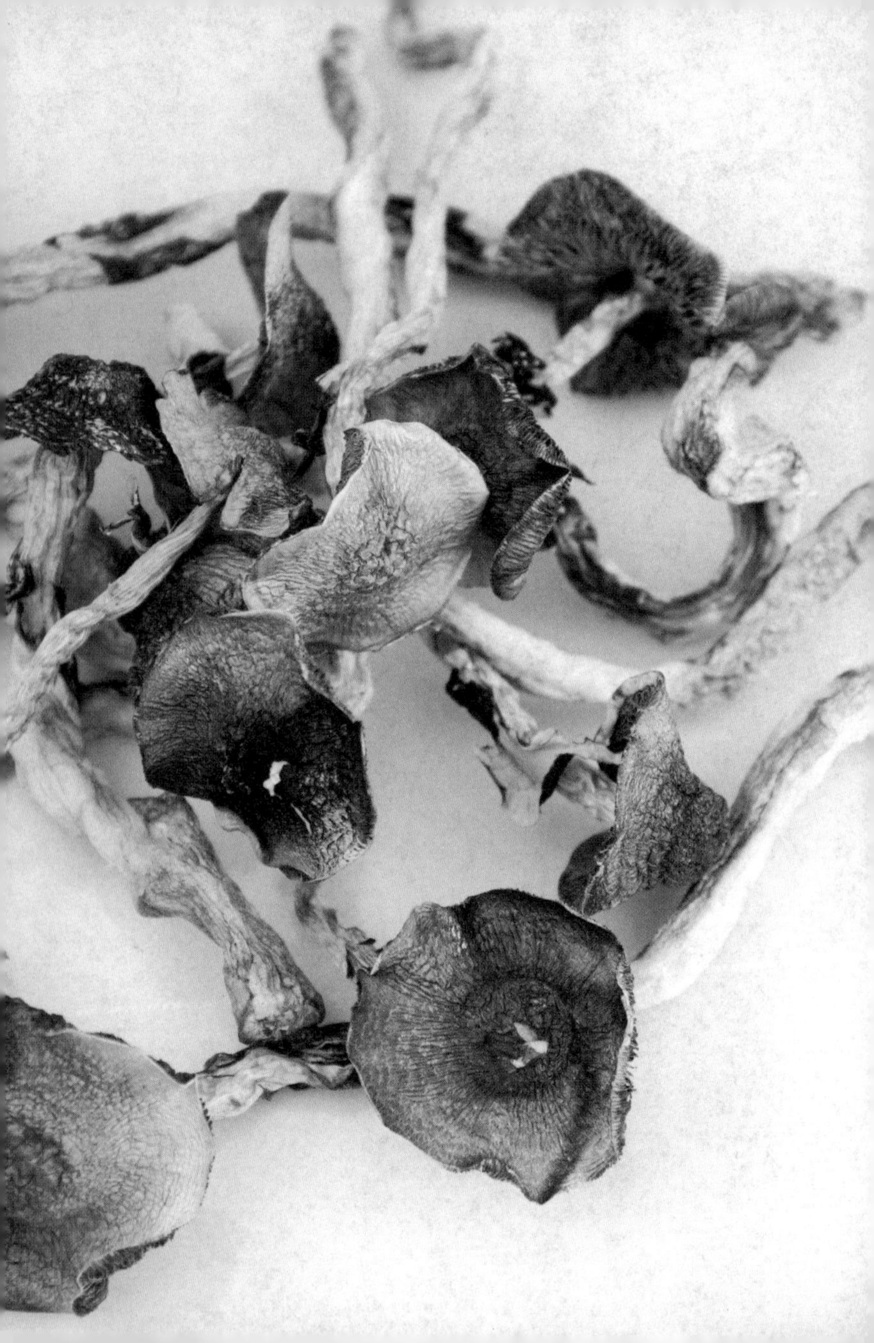

Simple Mushroom Powder

Ingredients

Dry Magic Mushrooms

Equipment

Coffee grinder, food processor, or blender

This is an easy one, but crucial for many of the baked goods you will find in later chapters of the guide.

First, gather (wild-picked or otherwise) roughly 20 dry-grams (or however much you wish, but let's start with 20 for the purpose of this book) of your favorite strain of psilocybin mushrooms. For consistency, we have decided to go with *Psilocybe cubensis*, but any other strain is just fine.

Next, you'll need a good coffee grinder or food processor. Make sure yours is of decent quality, as the fibrous stalks of the mushrooms can get caught up in the blades and ruin the motor of less powerful blenders if they're not dried to a cracker-like consistency.

For ease and accuracy a dehydrator is recommended. This piece of equipment will allow you to ensure that your mushrooms are fully and evenly dried. Other methods, such as using an oven or air drying are also viable, but the results may not be as consistent.

Simply grind your mushrooms until they form a fine powder. You can also add any spices you like to the mix. Just portion out however much mushroom powder you need and mix in the spices. For example, we have included a mushroom and pumpkin pie spice blend below.

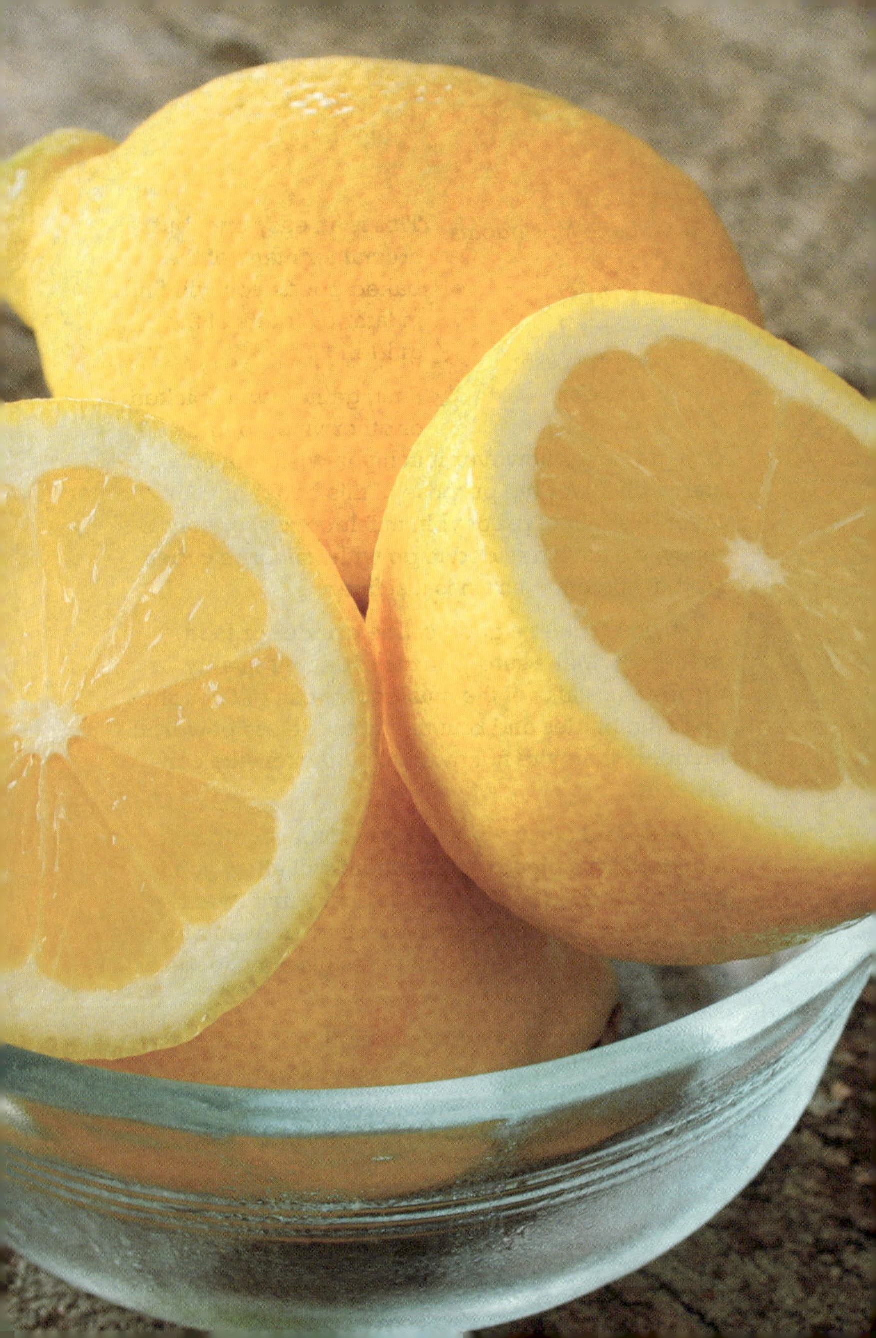

Lemon Tek

Lemon Tek is a popular method among psilocybin mushroom enthusiasts for consuming magic mushrooms. The technique involves using lemon or lime juice to pre-digest the mushrooms, potentially leading to a faster onset and more intense experience.

Ingredients

Dry Magic Mushrooms

1-2 large lemons

Equipment

Coffee grinder or mortar and pestle

Lemon juicer

Step 1: Grind Your Mushrooms

Start by finely grinding your dried psilocybin mushrooms to increase their surface area. A coffee grinder works well for this, but you can also use a knife or mortar and pestle. The finer the powder, the better the lemon juice can work on it. See the recipe for Simple Mushroom Powder on page 87 for more detailed instructions.

Step 2: Juice Your Lemons or Limes

Juice enough fresh lemons or limes to submerge the mushroom powder completely. Typically, one large lemon is enough for a single dose of mushrooms (1-2 grams). Strain the juice to remove any seeds or pulp.

Step 3: Mix Mushrooms with Lemon Juice

Place your ground mushrooms in a small, clean glass. Pour the freshly squeezed lemon or lime juice over the mushrooms until they are fully submerged. Stir the mixture gently to ensure all the mushroom powder is in contact with the acid.

Step 4: Let the Mixture Sit

Allow the mixture to sit for 20 to 30 minutes, stirring occasionally. The acid from the lemon juice will begin to break down the psilocybin into psilocin, a process that normally happens in the stomach. This pre-digestion can lead to a quicker and sometimes more intense psychedelic experience.

Step 5: Add Water (Optional)

After the waiting period, you can add a small amount of water to the mixture to dilute the intense lemon flavor if desired. This step is optional and based on personal preference.

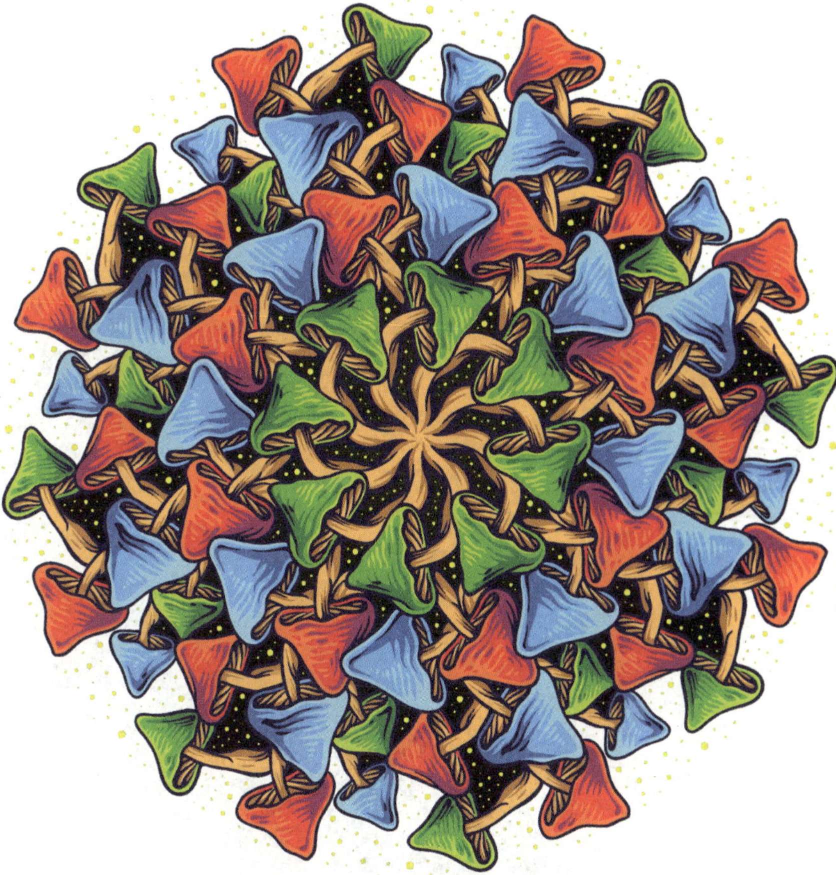

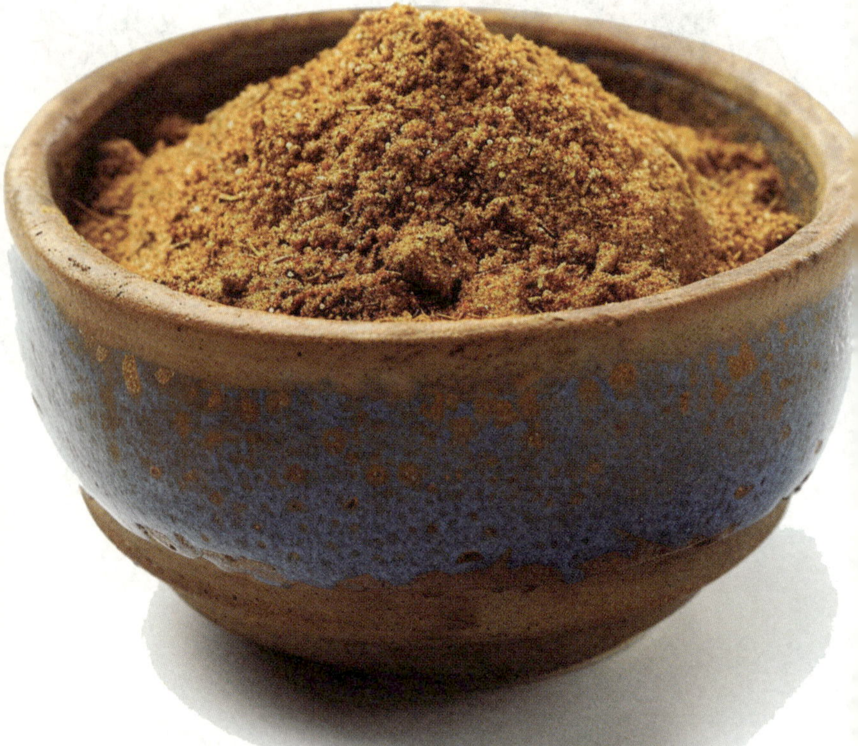

Mushroom/Pumpkin Pie Spice Blend

This simple spice blend was inspired by my grandmother's pumpkin pie recipe—a version of which is included later in the book. It is a subtle yet deliciously fun little mix of warm, nutty flavors, and, of course, psilocybin. This blend can also be combined with your favorite nuts and a little honey for a cosmically delicious snack. Enjoy!

Equipment

Coffee grinder, food processor, or blender

Ingredients

- *3 1/2 tablespoons of ground cinnamon*
- *2 1/4 teaspoons of ground ginger*
- *2 teaspoons of nutmeg*
- *2 teaspoons of ground allspice*
- *2 teaspoons of ground cloves*
- *4 grams of mushroom powder*

Preparation

Pulse your dry ingredients in a blender until the mixture is well, and thoroughly, combined. That's it!

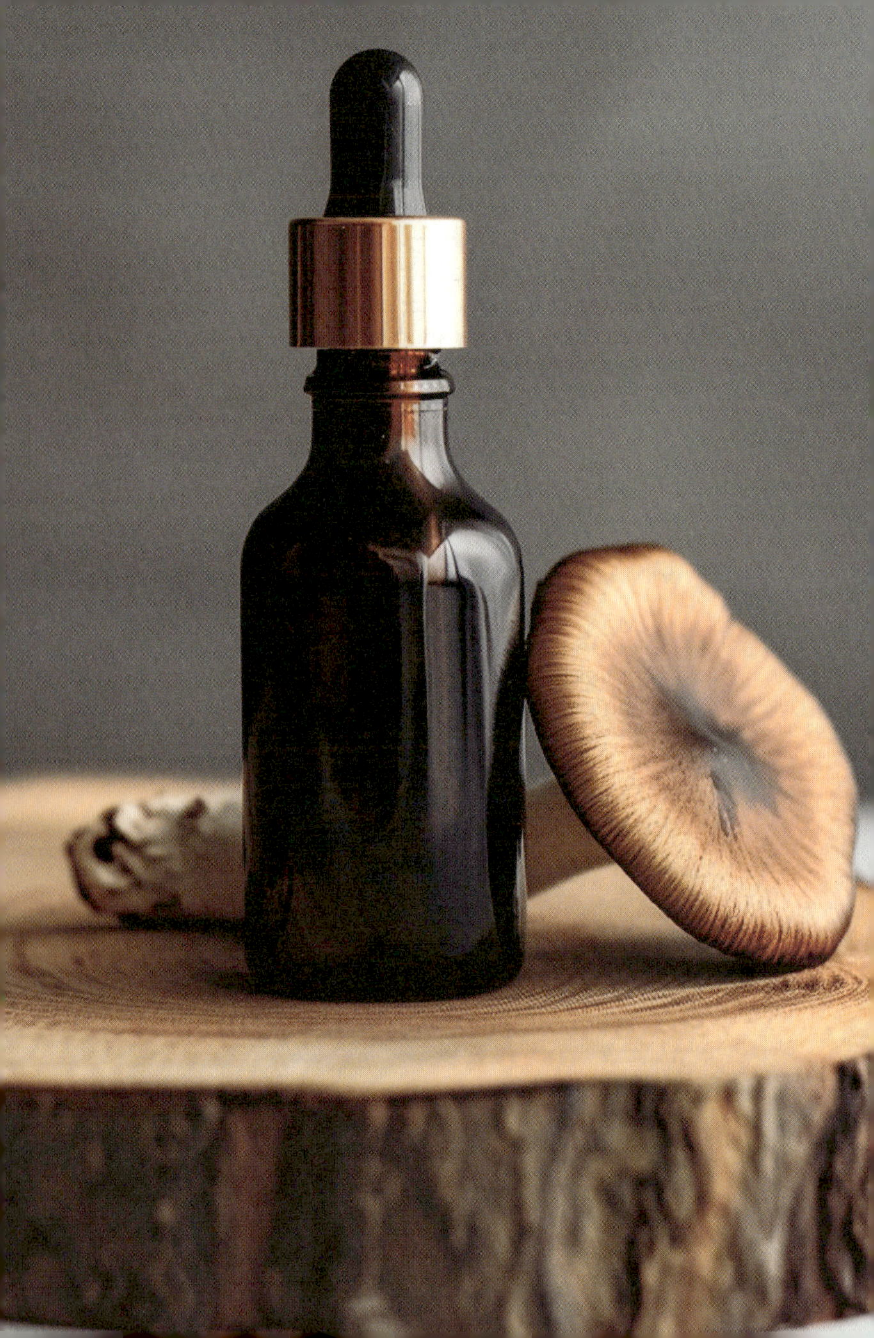

Basic Mushroom Elixir

This one is going to be a little more complex, but still easy. The main thing you'll need is patience as the entire process takes a few days. The result is undoubtedly worth the wait and will be a key part of many of the recipes to come.

Equipment

Coffee grinder, food processor, or blender

Two pint jars with lids

One medium-sized rubber band

A spoon or small spatula

Food processor

9x9 baking dish

100 ml beaker

2 oz Boston round bottle with scientific dropper

Small funnel

2 paper coffee filters (I like to use the cone shaped filters as they fit in your jars easier)

Ingredients

20 grams of your favorite fun-guys

750 ml bottle of good grain alcohol or vodka

Preparation

Alright, friends, let's get started. This particular recipe is going to read more like a science experiment than cooking, but the whole process is really fun. Bonus points to those of you who don a solid scientist costume while you work. We're going to start with a relatively mild elixir using 20 grams of dried mushrooms extracted into a final 40 ml solution. I've found that this gives you a moderate dose that's perfect for microdosing, or combining with teas, coffees, juices, and various other recipes that we will see later. You can, of course, scale this up for a stronger elixir if you find that this one is a little too mild for your needs. As always, the journey is yours, and once you have this process down pat, play around with it through trial and error until you find your favorite strength level.

Step One: Alcohol Extraction

Take your 20 grams of mushrooms and pulverize them by pulsing your grinder, the ideal consistency should be like very coarse sand; we don't want our mix to be too fine for this as you will end up with a cloudy solution if the particles are too small.

Next, place your freshly pulverized mushrooms in the pint jar you have ready to go. Now measure out 100 ml of grain alcohol using your beaker. Pour this over the mushrooms making sure that it just barely covers the top of your powder.

Now, securely fasten your lid onto the jar and then give it a few seconds of good, hard shaking. Go on, I know you can shake it a little harder, we want to be sure that our solution is thoroughly mixed. Once you've shaken the fun-guys until they're thoroughly mixed, and probably a little dazed and confused, set aside your jar. We're going to let this sit and soak for the next 48 hours (like I said, patience is key). In the meantime, feel free to have a handful of the nut and honey mix I mentioned earlier and take a load off.

Step Two: Evaporation and Concentration

And we're back! I hope you all enjoyed your break, now let's get this next step rolling. Grab your second pint jar, two coffee filters, and the rubber band. Double up the filters by placing one in the other. Slightly wet your coffee filters with some fresh cool water and then insert them into your second, clean jar. Leave just enough sticking out to fold over the top of the jar and then secure it with a rubber band.

Now, open the mushroom and alcohol mixture that you let sit for the last two days, and slowly pour it over your filters. Take a spoon or small spatula and gently tamp down the mixture periodically to ensure that it all fits. Once you've got everything inside the filters (go ahead and scoop out anything left in your jar) let the mixture drain into the new jar. Occasionally give the mix a gentle pat, or press, with your spoon/spatula until it has stopped dripping. Remove your filters full of mushroom material and set it aside, but don't discard it yet.

Now, bring over that 9x9 baking dish and pour your elixir into the pan. You will also want to grab your filter and give it a good squeeze to extract any remaining liquid into the pan. Once it is thoroughly wrung out you can go ahead and dispose of it (we like to compost ours). Now we must get ready to wait again. At this point, you're going to set the pan aside and let it rest, uncovered, while the alcohol evaporates. This can take a day or two—depending on how warm the room is and the alcohol content of the elixir. Periodically check on it, you're looking for it to form a slightly viscous solution.

Step Three: Bottling

Alright, it's been another few days, but we are finally at the finish line! Once it appears to be about right, gather a clean funnel and the 100 ml beaker. This is also a good time to take your spatula (recently washed) and gently stir the elixir. You want to break up any materials that have adhered to the bottom of the pan.

Next, place the funnel into the top of your beaker, and then gently pour the elixir from the pan and into the beaker. Once that is done, take note of the liquid volume in your beaker—we are aiming for a 40 ml solution. If you still have too much, simply let it sit out and continue to evaporate until you achieve the correct volume. If you have too little, just grab the bottle of grain alcohol, or vodka, that you used earlier, and pour some in until you have that 40 ml volume.

Okay, everyone, thanks for being patient with me—it's finally time to bottle your elixir! Set out your 2 oz Boston round bottle and place a funnel in the top. Slowly pour your elixir out of the beaker and into the funnel, taking care not to spill too much of it. Then, screw on the dropper lid. That's it, you're done!

Congratulations, my friends, you have successfully scienced the shit out of this!

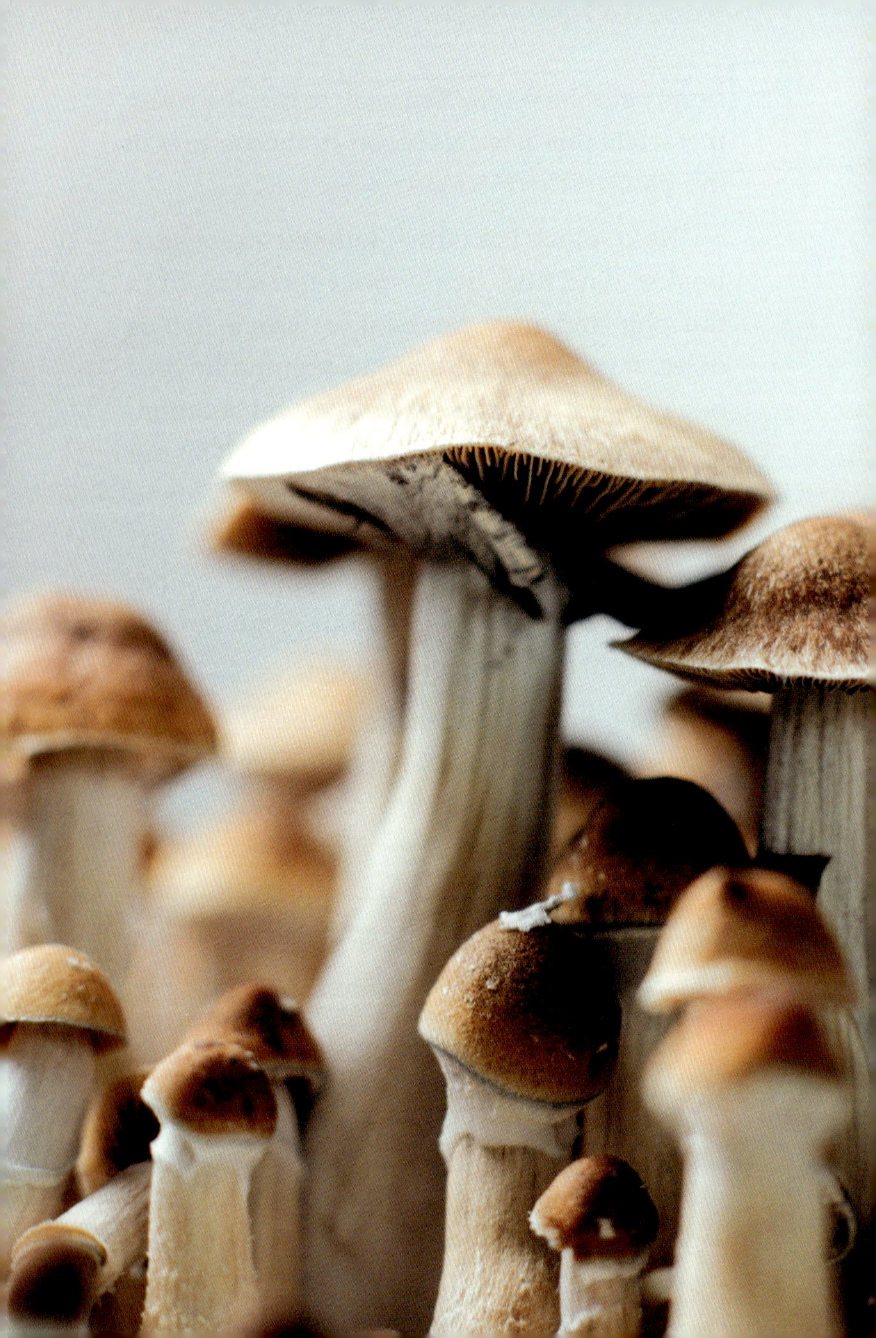

Paul Stamets' Original Blue Juice

Here, we have another very simple, but incredibly fun, extraction method. Originally from Paul Stamets, this cold-water extraction takes some time and patience, but is worth it in the end. You can use it in a variety of things, or just drink it as is. I like to add some lemon juice, ice, and a little sweetener, and make a big pitcher of Blue Lemonade (see page 105).

Note: This only works on fresh mushrooms. For some reason beyond my understanding, the psilocybin will not extract using this method with dried mushrooms.

Yield

Roughly 3 cups

Dose

2.6 grams per cup

Equipment

One 24 oz wide mouth mason jar with lid

Ingredients

3 cups of crushed ice

80 grams of fresh Magic Mushrooms

Preparation

The prep for this is quick and easy. Grab your 80 wet grams of fresh Magic Mushrooms and evenly, but not too finely, chop them. Scoop these into the mason jar and then begin adding in the ice. Continue to add crushed ice until the jar is completely full.

Place the full jar into the refrigerator. And now we wait—this takes a few days, so be patient.

Periodically check the jar and top it off with fresh ice one or two times.

After that, just let it sit and allow the ice to melt. As the ice melts, the cold water will extract the psilocybin from the fresh mushrooms.

Once the ice has completely melted you should be left with a jar full of blue/green juice. You can strain out the mushrooms, if you like, and put the juice in a clean jar, or not (it's completely fine either way, but the mushrooms get particularly soggy after a few days). From here, you can store it in the refrigerator for a few weeks or turn it into ice cubes.

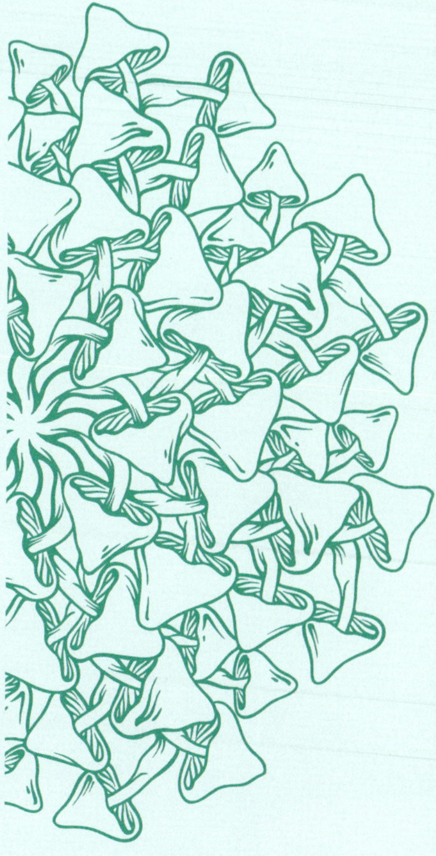

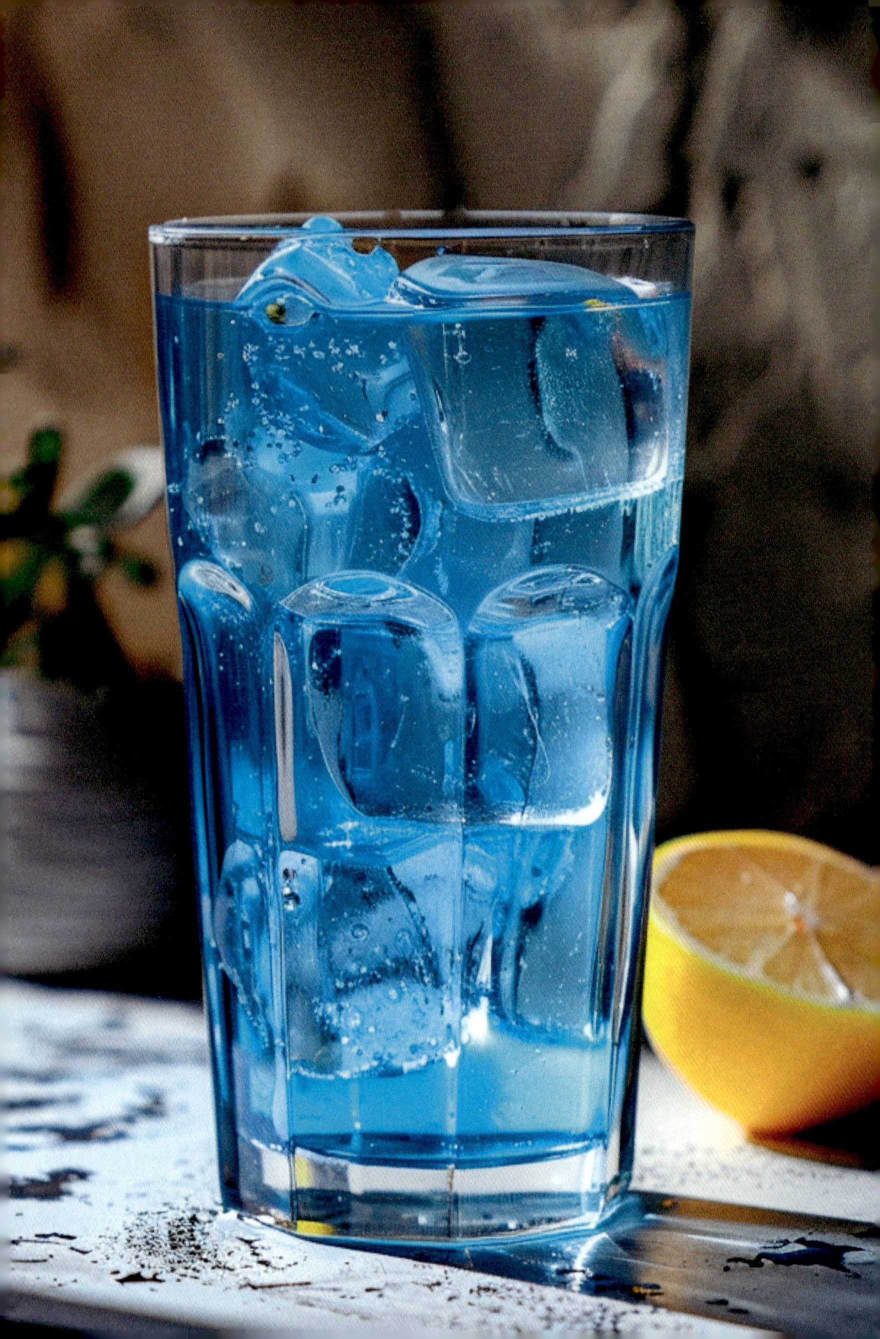

Stamets' Blue Lemonade

Stamets' Blue Lemonade is a quick, delicious, and refreshing drink that you can quickly put together using a few cups of blue juice, some sweetener, lemons, and ice.

The sweetness from the monk fruit (or any sweetener) is nicely complemented by the tart lemon juice. If you want to give it a little extra panache, throw in a bag of blue peaberry flower tea and watch it transform from deep blue to bright lavender. Mix up a pitcher and kick back on a hot day.

Yield

Roughly 6 servings

Dose

1 gram per serving

Ingredients

4 cups of water

3.5 cups of Stamets' Blue Juice

Juice of 6 large lemons

1 cup of monk fruit sweetener (or any other 1/1 sugar replacement)

Ice

Serving

Gather up some glasses, fill with crushed ice and pour. Serve this up to a group of close knit companions and prepare to go on a journey of self-discovery.

BLEND 'EM OR BREW 'EM

CHAPTER SIX

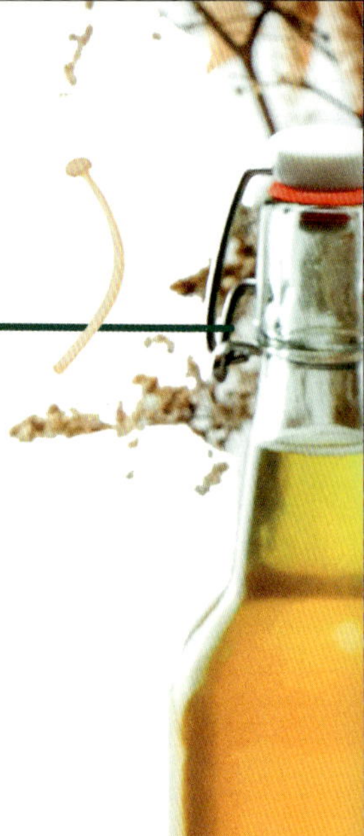

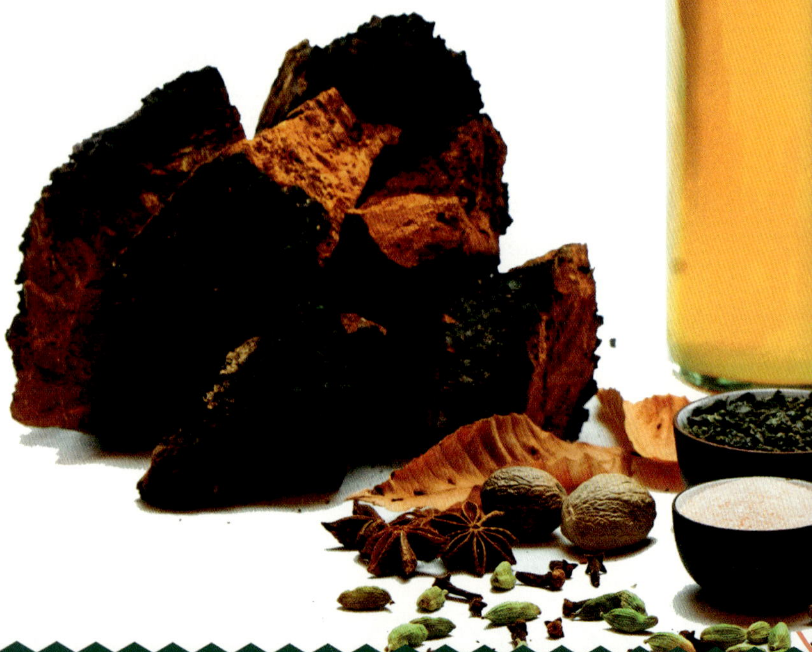

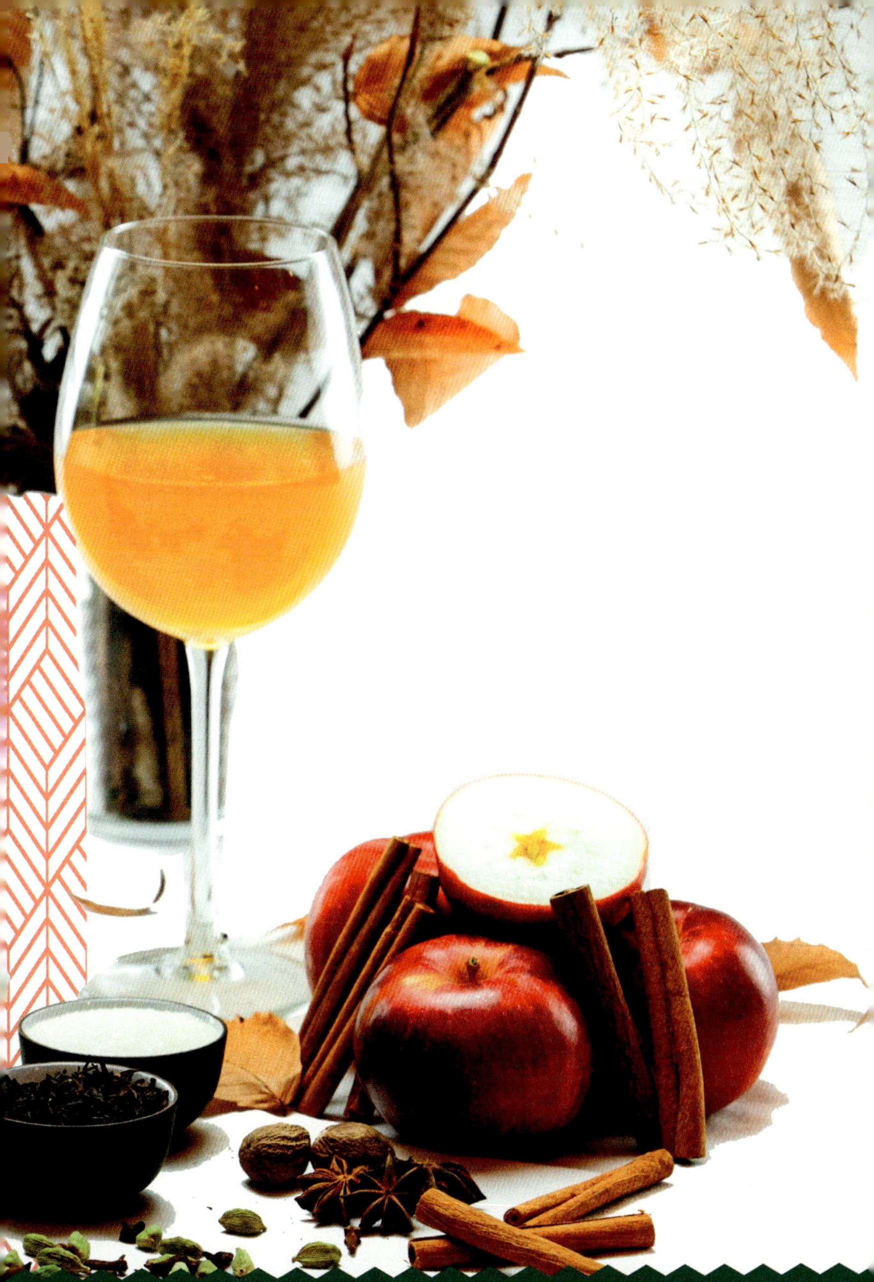

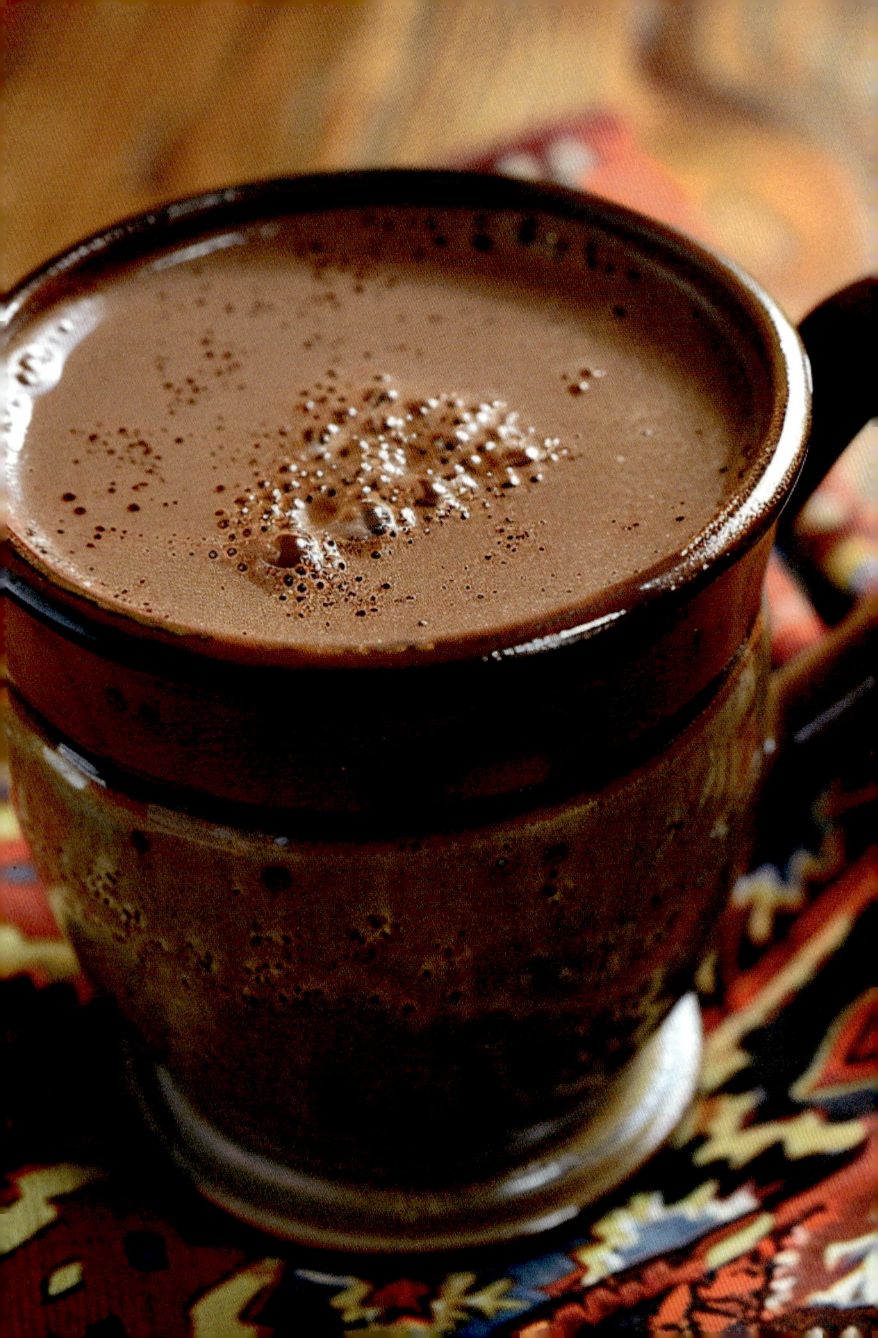

Ritual Cup Hot Chocolate

I was inspired to create this hot chocolate recipe based on my favorite Mexican hot chocolate from a little shop in San Pedro, California. It's made with real 99% dark chocolate, chipotle powder, a dash of cayenne pepper, and, of course, powdered funguys (we also added a dash of mentally stimulating lion's mane). The flavors mix wonderfully and will absolutely delight your taste buds. It is a strong, warming, and relaxing brew that I have always found will soften any hard edges, or relax me after a long, rough day. The dosage on this one is the highest of any of my recipes so please approach it carefully—this is NOT meant to be had before running out the door or driving. Be ready to sit down, stay home, (or take a nice walk) and have a long evening of contemplation, creation, and joy.

Yield

4 servings

Dosage

1.75 grams per serving

Ingredients

3 oz 99% dark chocolate

2 tablespoons unsweetened cocoa powder

3 tablespoons monk fruit sweetener (or any other 1/1 sugar replacement)

1/2 tablespoon cayenne pepper

1 tablespoon chipotle powder

1/2 teaspoon coarse sea salt

3 tablespoons lime juice

1 can coconut milk with liquid

7 grams powdered Magic Mushrooms

Preparation

Start by roughly chopping the dark chocolate. In a medium saucepan, warm the coconut milk over medium heat until it begins to simmer. Stir this occasionally. Add in the chopped dark chocolate and stir until it has fully dissolved. Add in the cocoa powder, cayenne pepper, monk fruit sweetener, and chipotle powder. Stir this until it is fully combined. Now add in the salt, powdered fun-guys, and lime juice. Reduce the heat to low and allow it to simmer while stirring constantly (we are going to use low heat, a little time, and acid to release some of the psilocybin). Continue this for about five minutes, if the liquid starts to get low you can top it off with a little water or milk substitute (or milk if you like dairy).

Serving

Get yourself a handful of mugs (I have some neat little mushroom mugs that I like to use), fill those babies up with your amazing hot chocolate mix, and then serve as is or top it off with some coco-whip (see page 140). Hand out a few cups to your troop of compatriots, and then prepare for a wildly relaxing evening and some sweet mental clarity (also probably some nifty visuals). Enjoy, my friends!

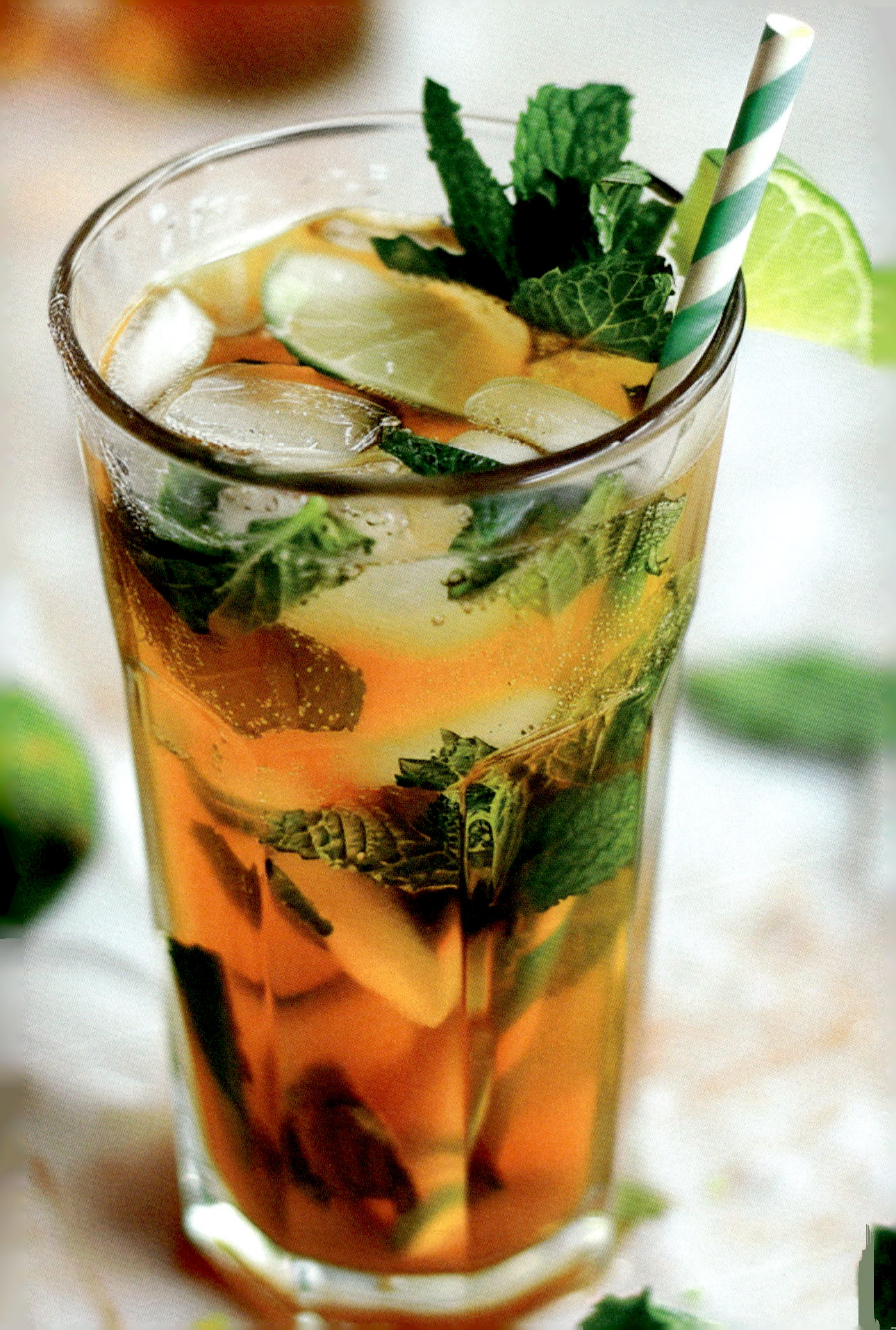

Refreshingly Cool Mint Lime Tea with Honey

This wonderfully refreshing, and slightly funky, mint tea was invented by my friend Branden on a particularly balmy 91-degree day. It's a simple, but delicious summer (or anytime) refresher that's perfect to enjoy with a group of friends around the pool or on a sunny back porch. The effects of a single glass are not too strong, and tend to provide you with a nice body high with increased clarity and creativity. Combined with the slightly caffeinated green tea, this will perk you up and get your mind ready to enjoy a lovely afternoon of sun and fun. Pour out a few glasses and be prepared for a journey of discovery with your closest friends.

Yield

8 servings

Dose

0.5 grams per serving

Ingredients

3 bags of herbal mint tea (we like to use Moroccan mint from Trader Joe's)

2 large bags of green tea (any brand is fine, and feel free to substitute regular for decaf)

1 oz of your favorite honey

8 cups of fresh, cold water

8 ml Mushroom Elixir (you may add more but we find that this gives you a nice, but not overwhelming, dose)

1 lime, juiced

Fresh mint for garnish

Ice

Brewing

Bring the cold water to a boil in your kettle, or simply a pot if no kettle is on hand. Once it's ready to go, pour the hot water into your pitcher, then add in your tea. Let it steep according to the package instructions, or roughly 3 minutes. Once your tea is done steeping, go ahead and remove your tea bags. I like to set them to the side to cool for a few minutes before squeezing out the remaining liquid. After that, discard your bags.

Now, add the honey and stir using a long spoon until it has fully dissolved in the tea. Set your hot tea in the refrigerator to cool for 2-4 hours. Once cooled, take your lime and juice it; you can use a lime juicer if you like, or go the easy route (my preferred method) and just squeeze them directly in the pitcher. Give it a quick stir to mix in the juice. Now, measure out your 8 ml of mushroom elixir and stir that in as well. Remember, you can always add more to achieve your desired strength, or less for that matter, but as always be mindful of your dosing. Stir a little more and place the tea back in the refrigerator to cool.

This should be stored in the refrigerator and your tea will last several days without any noticeable loss of potency. This cannot be said for storing the tea at room temperature as psilocybin tends to break down quickly at room temperature.

Serving

Gather up a few glasses, as many as needed, and fill them with ice. I like to use crushed ice. Take your fresh mint, give it a quick washing, and pluck off any brown and dried up leaves (you can let these dry in the sun and powder them). Gently bruise your mint, and then place it into the glass. Next, grab another lime and slice a few thin rounds off it. Make some quick cuts into the round so the lime can sit on the rim of your glass.

Pour a glass of tea, and stick that fancy little lime slice on there for garnish. Voila! You've got yourself a refreshingly psychedelic glass of tea to enjoy on a hot day!

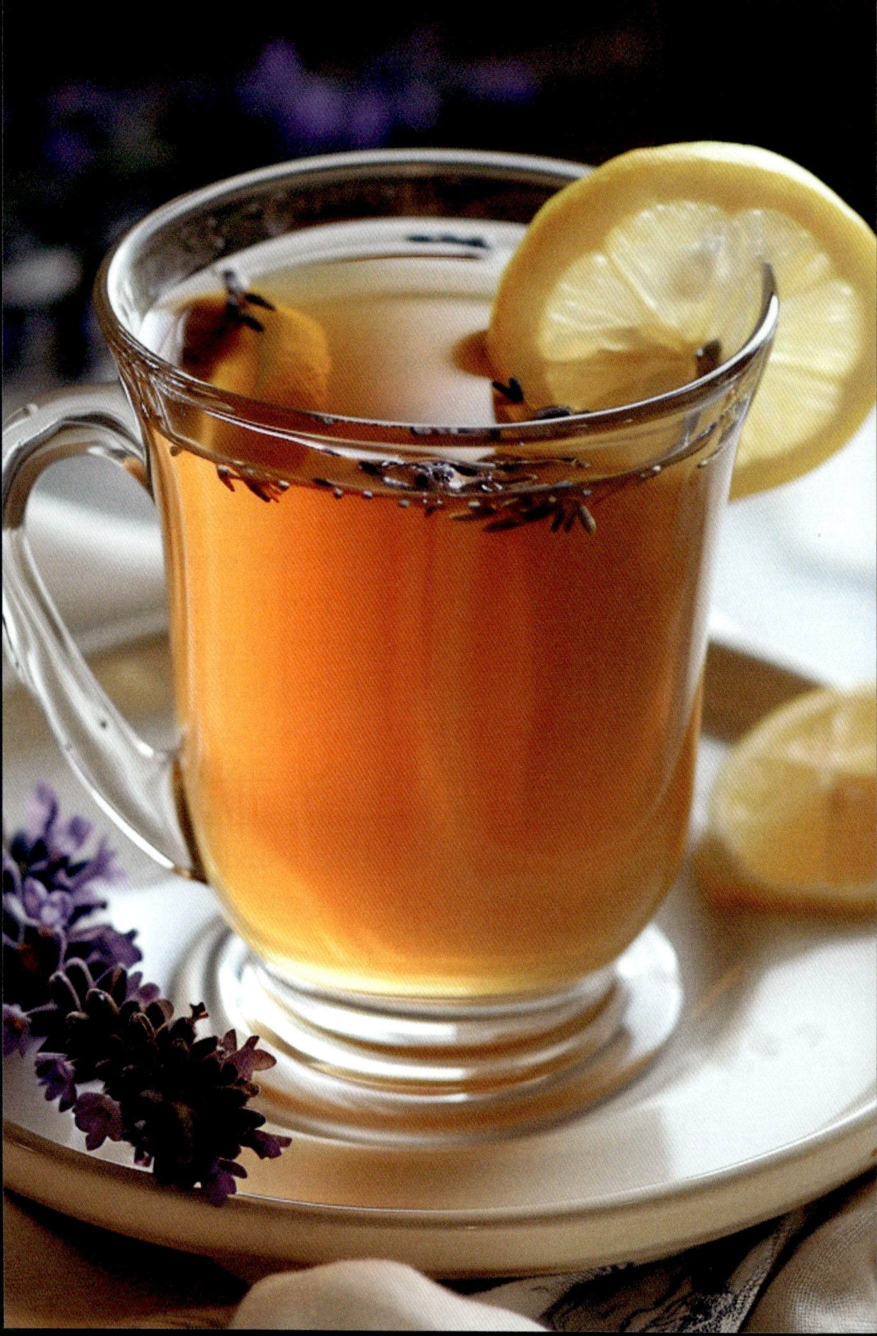

Mushroom Toddy with Dried Lavender and Wildflower Honey

The inspiration for this soul-warming tea came to me on a dreary fall afternoon that needed a little brightening up. The lavender combines scrumptiously with wildflower honey, smoky Scotch, and crisp oolong tea, topped off with a slice of vibrantly tart lemon. It has just enough fun-guys in the mix to give you an interesting and groovy state of consciousness, while still being able to navigate through your day. Excellent when shared with like-minded souls during a long paint-party or by yourself and a good book (no wandering words here, unless you decide to spice up the dose).

Yield

4 servings

Dose

1 gram per serving

Ingredients

4 cups of cool fresh water

4 bags of your favorite oolong tea, or enough loose-leaf tea for four

4 tablespoons of locally sourced wildflower honey

2 tablespoons of dried lavender

4 grams of cracker-dry mushrooms, roughly chopped and divided into one-gram servings

1 lemon, cut and quartered

8 oz of Scotch divided into fourths, I like to use Glenfiddich 12-year-old Single Malt (I know, looking like Snooty McGhee over here)

Optional Items

A fancy looking mushroom tea pot and little mushy-shaped cups for serving (completely unnecessary but oh-so-satisfying).

Brewing

As with all teas, this is pretty simple. Bring your water to a boil, or heat until the kettle toots. Next, there are two options—first is my preferred method. Whip out that fancy, little, fungus-impersonating teapot, and pour the water in. Now, throw in your four tea bags and the infuser—loaded up with dried lavender and mushrooms. Let the tea steep for five to ten minutes before removing the bags and lavender diffuser.

While that steeps, grab your mushy-cups and add in the scotch, pouring just 2 oz per cup. Then, squeeze some fresh lemon into each. Let this sit while the tea finishes steeping. Once the tea has steeped, gather your friends and pour out a few cups. Feel free to mix in the honey at this point, or leave it out for a sugar free experience. Lastly (and this part is absolutely mandatory) take a sip, hug your friends, or open that book, and start to relax. You're in for a fun time!

For the other method, the first few steps are the same, but here, we are going to dispense with the fancy, and totally necessary, but not, teapot. Instead, simply add 1 gram of roughly chopped mushrooms, 1/2 tablespoon of lavender, and a tea bag to each cup. Pour in hot water, add the scotch, and lemon, then let steep for five or ten minutes. From here, you can fish out the mushrooms and lavender with a spoon, or just let it be (I vote for the latter option). Remove the bags and serve with or without honey. Enjoy!

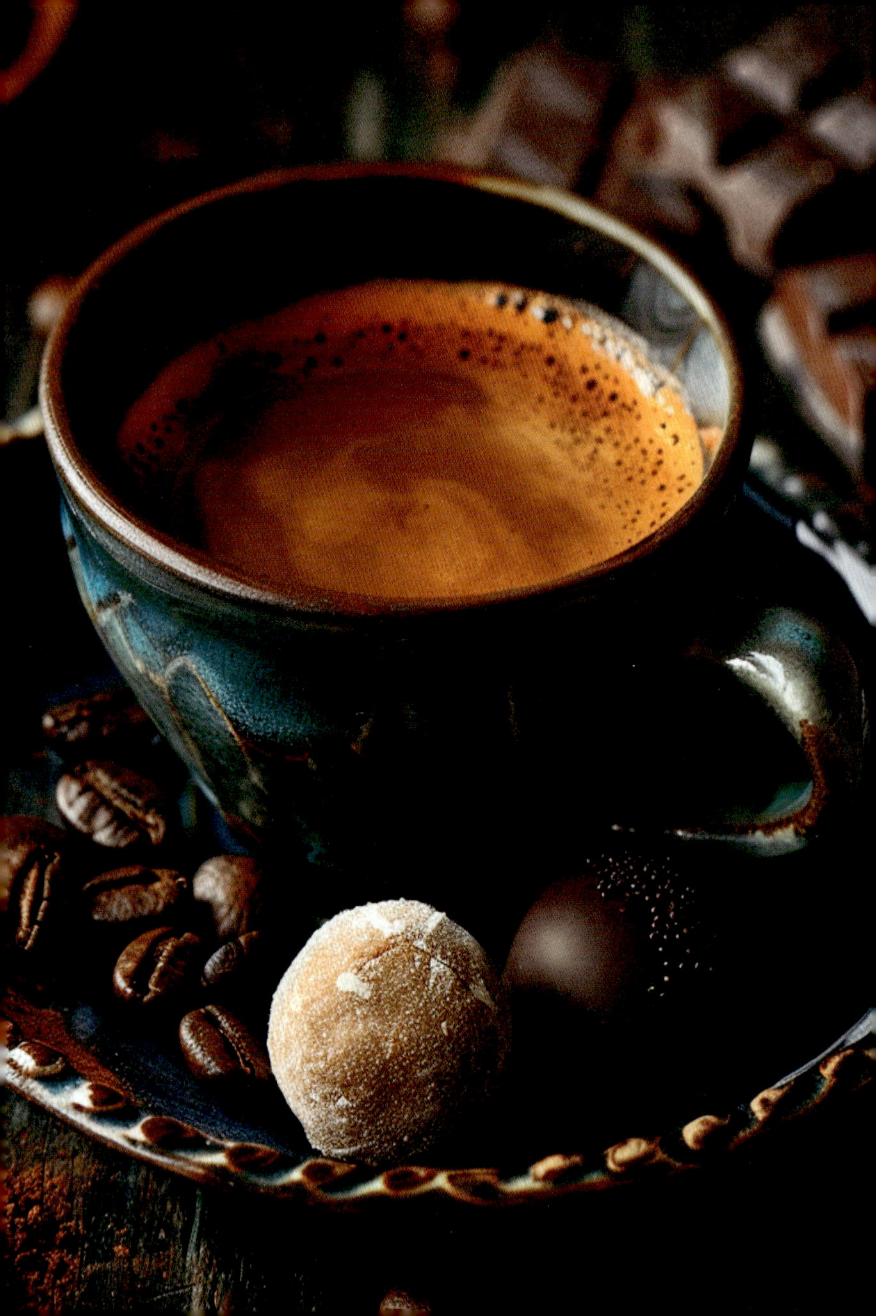

Cubensis Coffee to Start Your Day (Microdose Version)

Coffee and cubensis? What an absolutely delightful little combination to get your mind going and ready for a long day of inspiration and creativity. This is a simple recipe that's mostly (remember, I'm kind of a diva) devoid of fuss and flair, but is still delicious. I like to use a French press for just me, and a regular pot for groups of four or more. Although the coffee you use doesn't make a huge difference, it's best with freshly ground beans (Three Bears Coffee in Knoxville, Tennessee roasts some amazing beans), and a little almond milk—with just a spoonful of monk fruit sweetener and a cinnamon stick for stirring. Pour yourself a slightly steamy cup and prepare to greet the day.

Yield

5 servings

Dose

.20 grams per serving

Equipment

6 Cup French press

Sunshine (unless you're a night owl, then moonlight will do)

Ingredients

4 cups of cool, fresh water

1 1/2 tablespoon fresh ground coffee per cup of water

2 teaspoons of unsweetened almond milk

1 teaspoon of monk fruit sweetener or honey (whichever you prefer)

4 cinnamon sticks

1 gram of powdered Psilocybe cubensis

Optional Items

Some neat, little, mushroom coffee cups

Brewing

Bring your water up to a temperature that's just above a slow simmer, but not boiling as we don't want the coffee to become bitter from overheating. Grind your fresh beans and add those into the French press along with the powdered mushrooms. Pour over the hot water and let it fill your press. After that, put the lid on and let the coffee and mushroom steep for around 5 minutes before you press the plunger down.

Serving

While that steeps, gather some cups and add sweetener and cinnamon sticks. Now, plunge that plunger! Done? Pour in the coffee and add your favorite almond milk, or other non dairy creamer, and give it a quick stir with the cinnamon stick. Set aside the used coffee grounds to use for our Cubensis Coffee Cake (see page 161), and enjoy with a few other beautiful spirits, or just by your ever-so-amazing self.

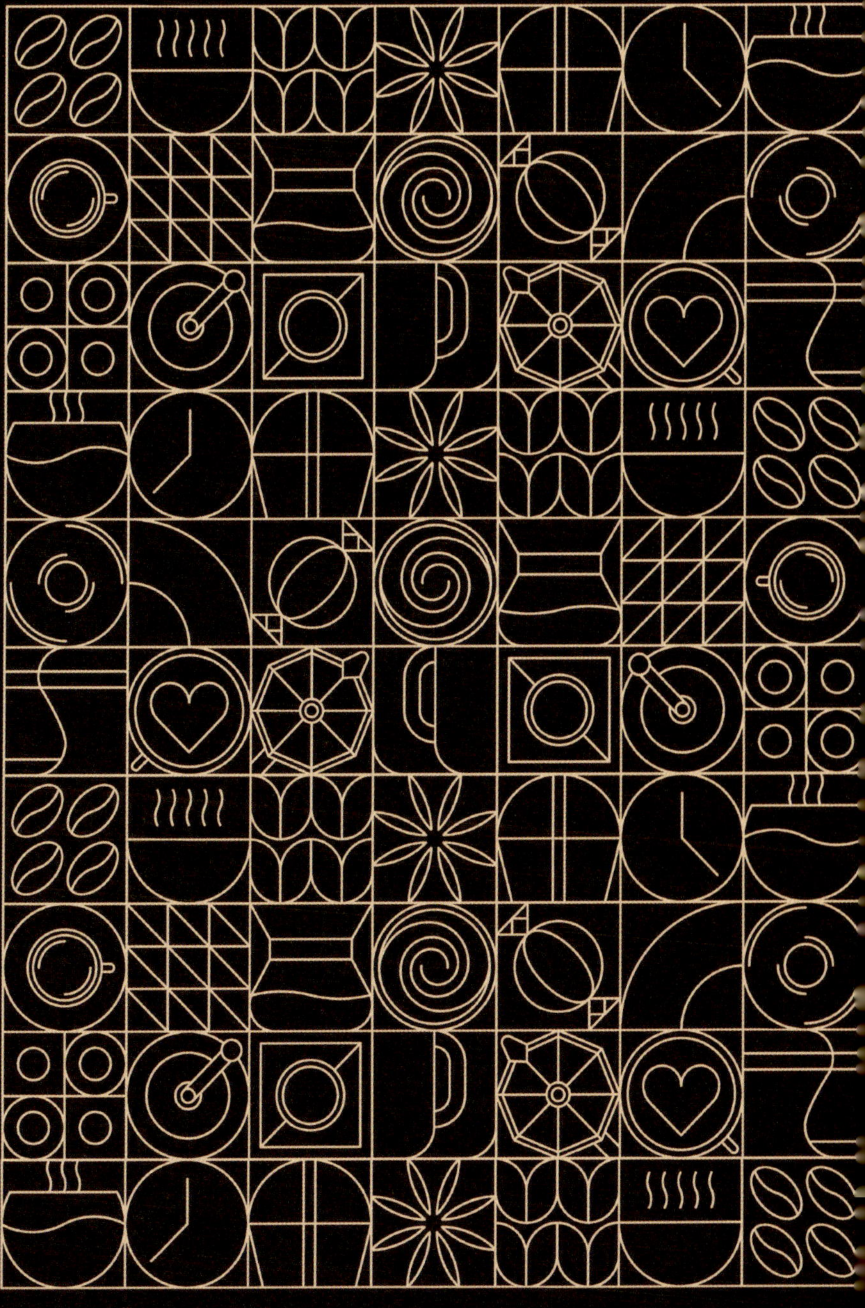

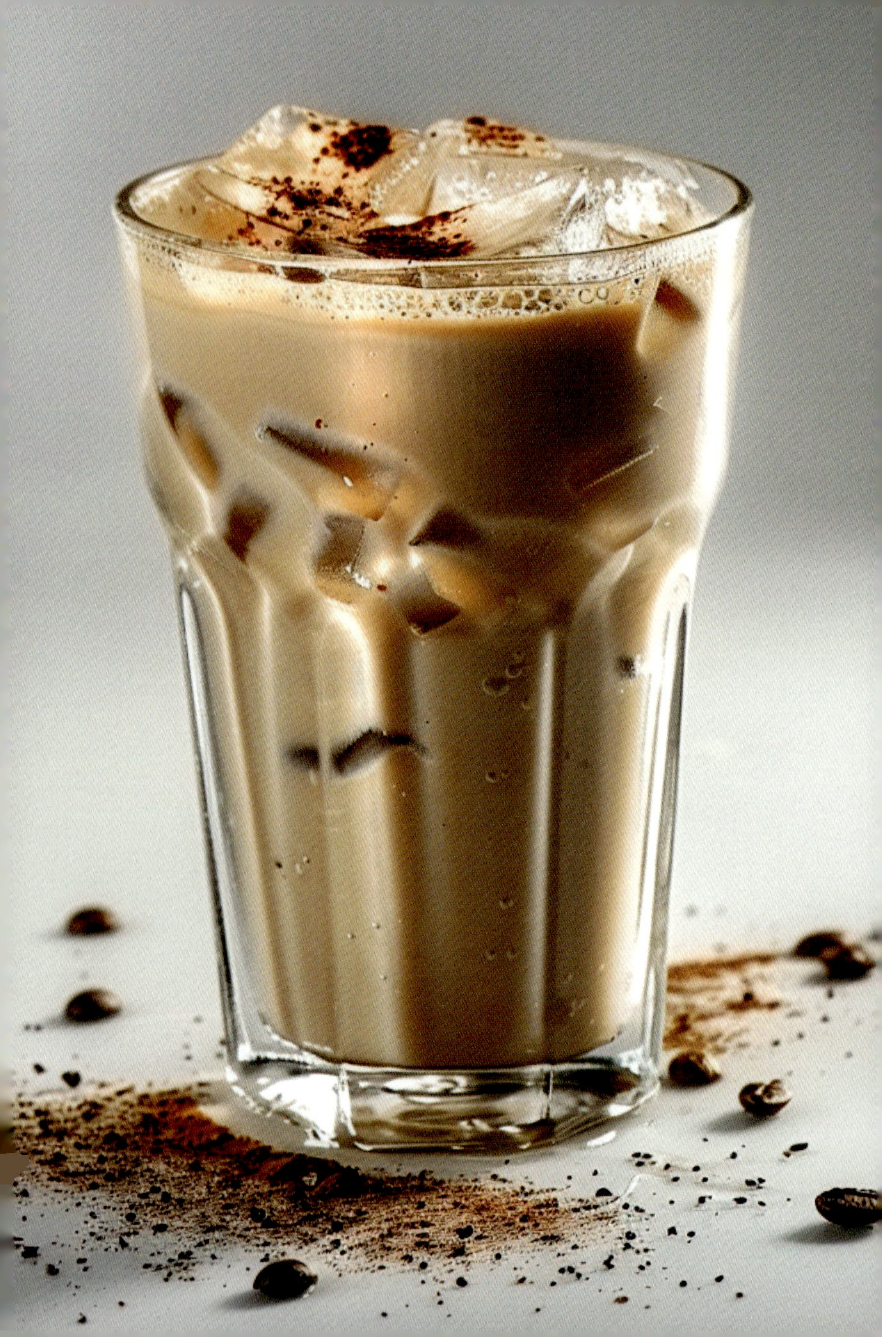

Cubensis Cold Brew for Creative Mornings (Low-Dose Version)

Who said coffee has to be hot to spark the imagination? Not I, said the cat. This Cubensis Cold Brew is your ticket to a chilled, inspired start to any day, blending the rich, earthy tones of your favorite coffee with a touch of psychedelic wonder. Perfect for sipping as you watch the sunrise or under the stars if you're the nocturnal artist type. Freshly ground coffee is our muse, and a dash of almond milk with a whisper of sweetener makes this concoction just divine.

Yield

4 servings

Dose

1 gram per serving

Equipment

A large mason jar (or any jar with a lid)

Sunshine for the brew, moonlight for the muse

Ingredients

4 cups of cold, filtered water

6 tablespoons of coarsely ground coffee

4 grams of powdered Psilocybe cubensis (for that sprinkle of magic)

2 teaspoons of unsweetened almond milk (or your creamer of choice)

1 teaspoon of monk fruit sweetener or honey

4 cinnamon sticks (for a hint of spice and everything nice)

Brewing

In your most cherished mason jar, mix the coarsely ground coffee with the powdered mushrooms—this is where the magic begins. Gently pour in the cold water, stirring softly to ensure everything is nicely blended. Seal the jar with love and let it sit out in the sunshine (or moonlight, for our night owls) for about 12 to 24 hours. The longer it brews, the deeper the flavors and the more profound the morning muse.

Serving

Once your brew has reached its peak potential, strain it to keep only the liquid (a fine mesh sieve or cheesecloth works wonders here). In your chosen mushroom-themed mug, add a teaspoon of your preferred sweetener, a dash of almond milk for creaminess, and a cinnamon stick for that final, aromatic flourish. Pour over your cold brew concoction, stir gently with the cinnamon stick, and prepare to greet the day (or night) with a soulful sip of creativity.

Remember, this cold brew is not just a drink; it's a morning ritual to awaken the senses and the inner muse. Enjoy it in solitude as you pen down your thoughts, or share the magic with fellow dreamers. Here's to starting your day on a note of inspiration and a touch of whimsy. Cheers to your health and to the endless possibilities that await.

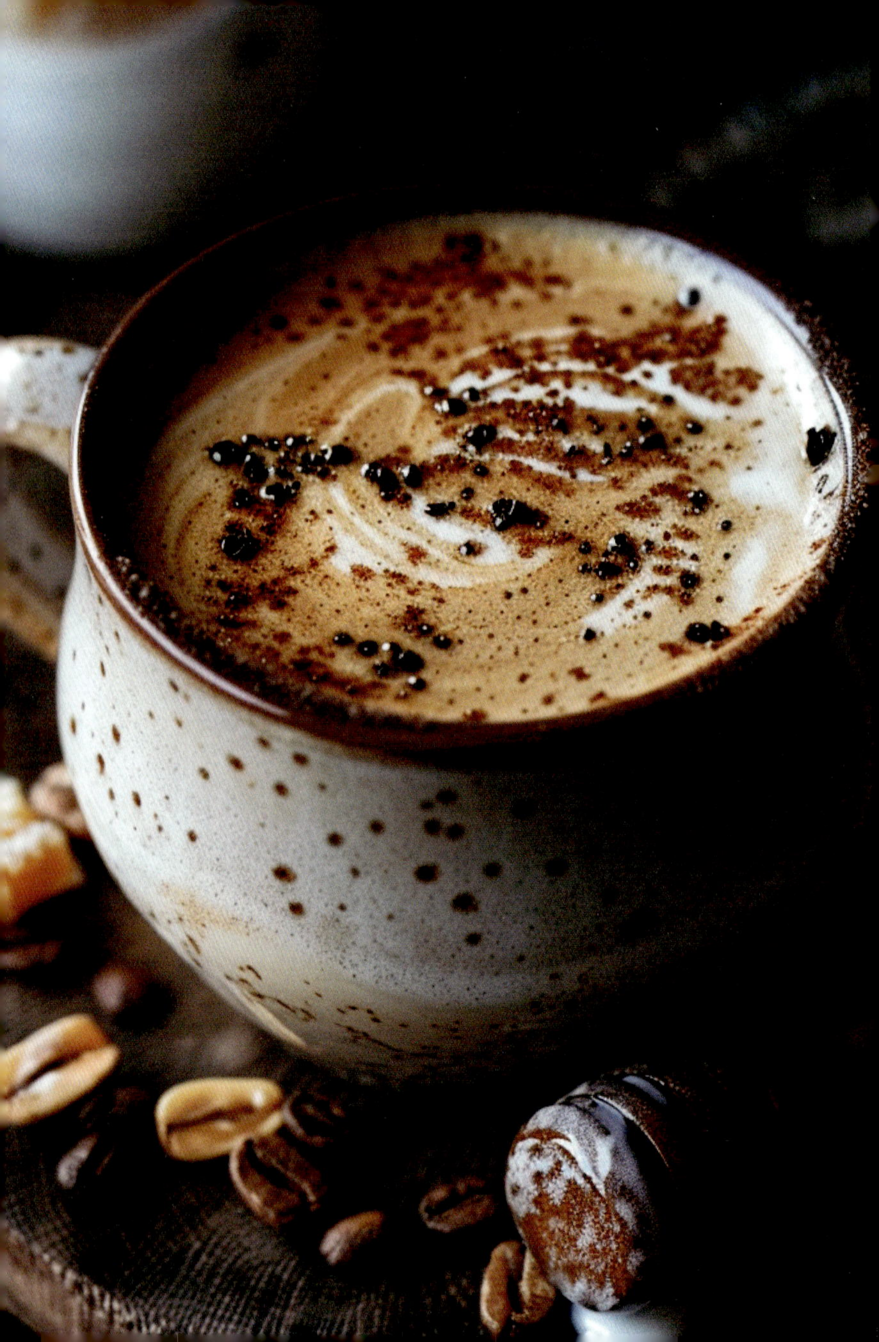

Star-Side Fungi-ccinos with Honey and Oat Milk

My personal take on a favorite treat of mine; this fun-guy infused frap is perfect for a quick pick-me-up on a busy day. With just enough caffeine to get you going, and a not-too-strong dose of psilocybin, you'll be ready to power through your daily routine. The flavors of the oat milk, espresso, and dark chocolate, will soothe your taste buds and liven up your creative side. I like to serve it with a reusable flexi-straw and a dollop of homemade coco-whip (see our Key Lime Pie recipe on page 153). Go the extra mile and grate a little more chocolate on top for some fancy points.

Yield

2 servings

Dose

1 gram per serving

Ingredients

- *2 cups oat milk*
- *1/2 teaspoon vanilla extract*
- *1 1/2 tablespoon instant espresso (I like Megdalia D'Oro, it's easy to find at most grocery stores)*
- *1/4 teaspoon salt (don't leave this out)*
- *2 tablespoons monk fruit sweetener or honey*
- *4 ml of Mushroom Elixir*
- *4 oz of good, dark chocolate (We use Endangered Species 88% dark. Not only is it delicious, but proceeds go towards conservation of threatened and endangered animals.)*
- *4 cubes of frozen Cubensis-Coffee (Or just ice)*

Optional Items

- *Chilled mugs fresh from the freezer*

Preparation

Oh look, a coffee drink that doesn't require boiling water! This here's an easy one, folks. Pour your oat milk (or substitution) into the blender. Next, add the vanilla extract, instant espresso, chocolate, and salt. Give the blender a few quick pulses to combine the ingredients before adding in your frozen coffee cubes or ice. Blend until you have a nice smoothie-like texture. Lastly, add in your 4 ml of Mushroom Elixir, and pulse 3 or 4 times until thoroughly combined.

Serving

Simply fill each glass nearly to the brim, stirring occasionally to ensure an even distribution of slush. Now, add a little (or large) blob of coco-whip and, most importantly, grate some more chocolate on there. Say it with me, chocolate, chocolate, chocolate! All that's left is to sip and enjoy while basking in your own chocolatey, shroomy glory.

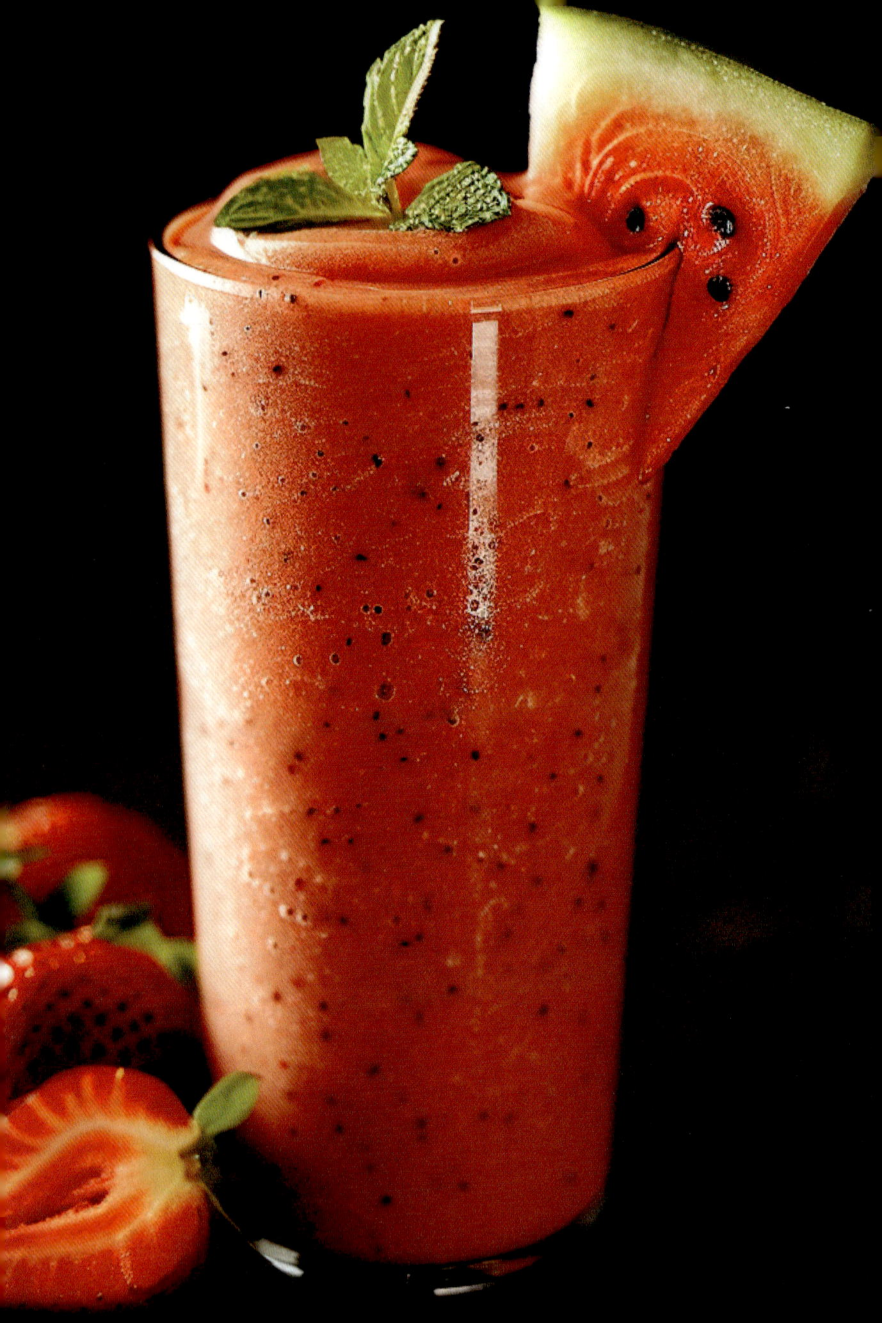

Kickin' Super Berry Watermelon and Lion's Mane Smoothie

This smoothie is an adaptation of my mother's recipe from many, many summers ago (we won't say how many). It is wonderfully flavorful and packed with tons of antioxidants. The addition of the lion's mane mushrooms pairs well with our fun-guys as they are thought to further enhance the neuro-regenerative and cognitive enhancing traits of psilocybin. It is also just yummy, plain and simple. I really like the way the tart, black cherries play off the strawberries and fresh watermelon. Those of you worried about the flavor being heavy on the fungus, never fear, you can barely taste the lion's mane (which has a mild mineral flavor on its own) and the Mushroom Elixir is fully covered by the explosion of fresh, fruity greatness.

Yield

4 servings

Dose

1 gram per serving

Ingredients

1 cup frozen black cherries, roughly chopped (this helps with blending)

1 cup fresh strawberries

1 cup frozen blueberries

1 cup fresh watermelon

1/2 cup fresh lime juice

1/2 cup crushed ice

8 ml Mushroom Elixir

Optional Items

Fancy, little, cocktail umbrellas

3 grams of fresh lion's mane mushroom (omitted if not available)

Preparation

Gather your various fruits and begin adding it to the blender. Starting with the frozen cherries, pulse the blender until the cherries are broken up into small pieces. Next, add in your frozen blueberries and repeat the pulsing process (pulse, pulse, pulse!). After that, add fresh fruit in any order, as well as the crushed ice, and juice. Lastly, we are going to blend in the Lion's Mane mushroom and fun-guy elixir. Continue to blend until your smoothie reaches the desired consistency.

Serving

The absolute best (i.e. fanciest) way to serve these delicious little smoothies is in four, large margarita glasses. Pour out even portions, and top with a lime garnish and cocktail umbrella. Share this easy summer refresher with your chosen life partners and kick your feet up!

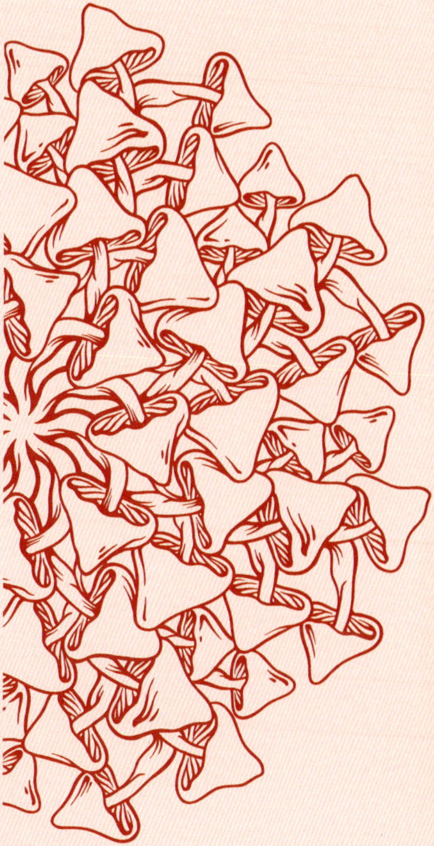

FANTASTIC TREATS & HOW TO MAKE THEM

CHAPTER SEVEN

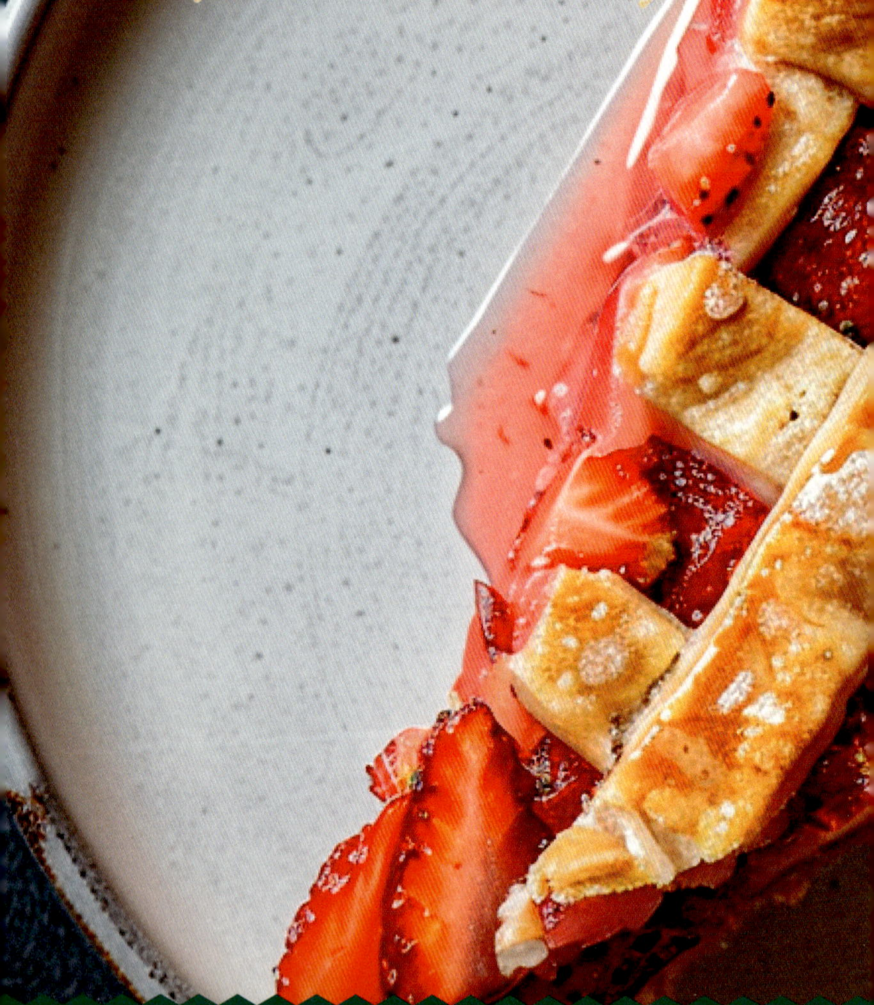

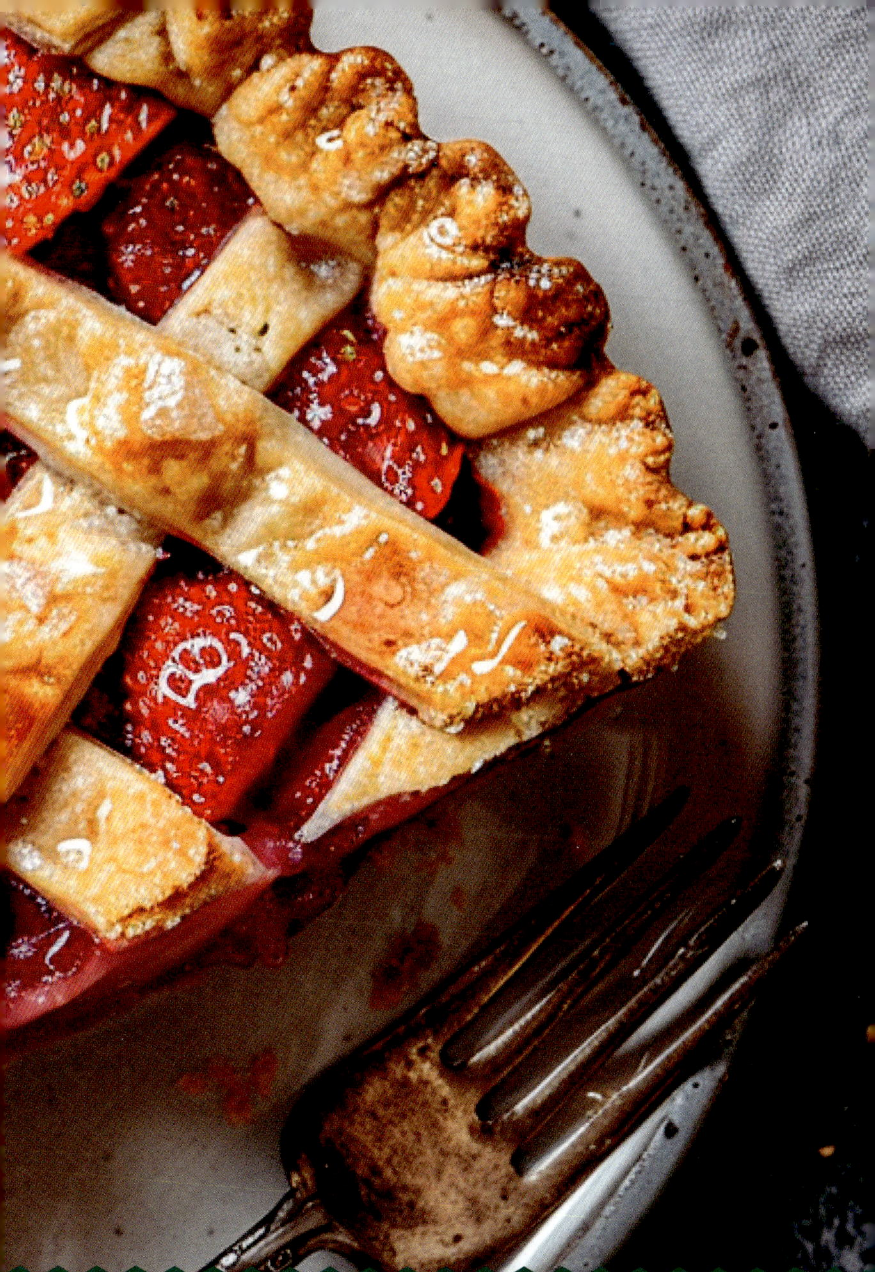

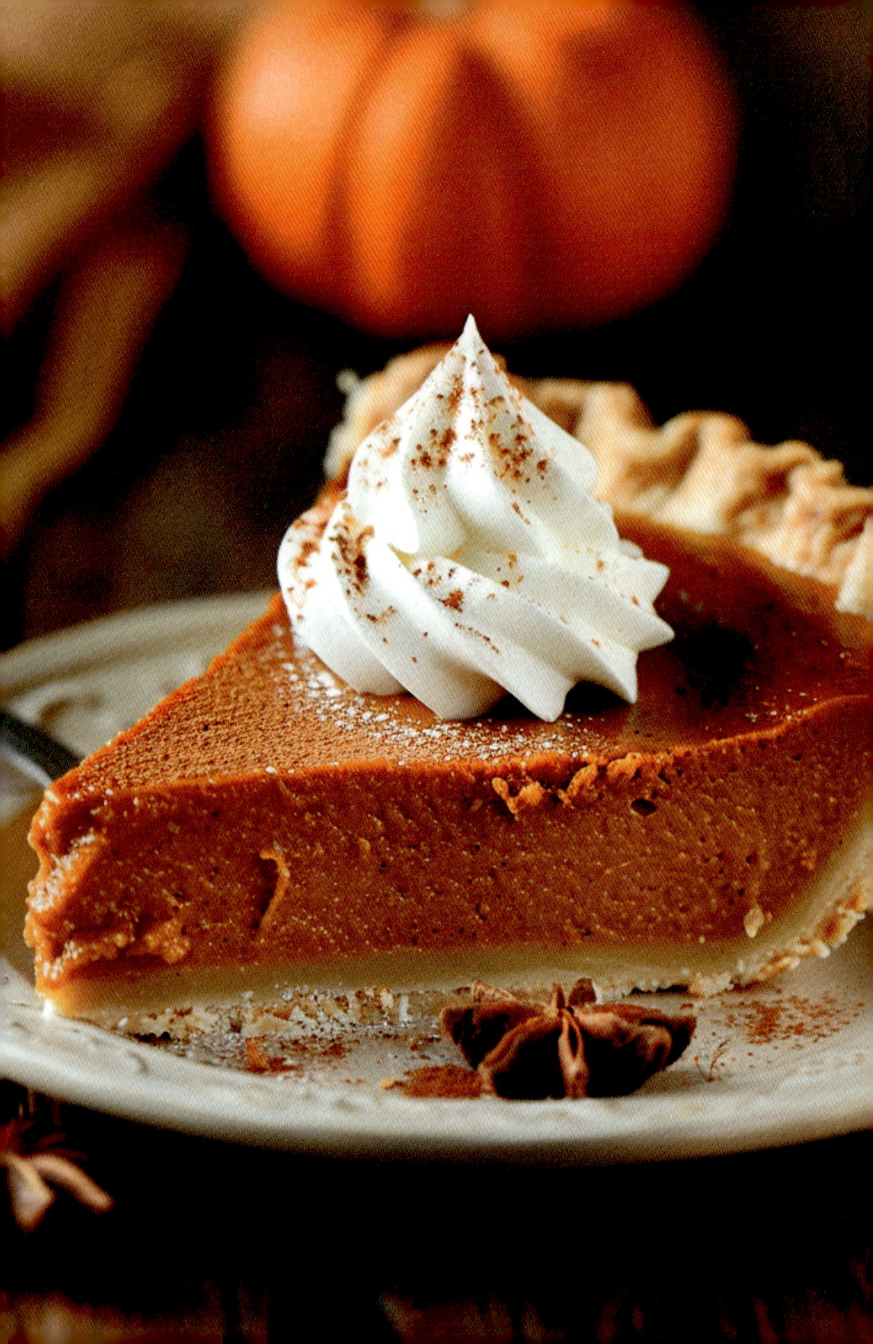

Perfectly Pumpkiny Mushroom Pie

How better to start off our desserts than with a classic pumpkin pie? This warm, fall time treat is delightfully satisfying, with its flaky and buttery gluten-free crust, warmly spiced filling, and, naturally, a dash of magic from our fun-guy friends. This recipe is based off of my grandmother's pumpkin pie, which has stood unchanged since at least 1952. Pair it with an ice cold glass of your favorite milk, or milk substitute, and a whopping dollop of coco-whip for an out-of-this-world treat.

Yield

8 servings

Dose

0.5 grams per serving

Gluten Free Pie Crust

1 ten inch gluten-free pie crust

1 1/3 cups organic gluten-free all-purpose flour

1/2 teaspoon salt

1/2 cup chilled organic vegetable shortening

1 large egg

4 tablespoons ice water

Pie Filling

1 cup monk fruit sweetener

2 eggs

15 oz organic pumpkin purée

1 1/2 cup coconut cream solids fully melted

Magically Mushroomed Pumpkin Pie Spice

2 teaspoons ground cinnamon

1/2 teaspoon ground ginger

1/4 teaspoon nutmeg

1/4 teaspoon ground allspice

1/4 teaspoon ground cloves

4 grams of mushroom powder

Coco-whip Topping

1 can full-fat coconut cream (chilled)

1 tablespoon maple syrup

1/2 teaspoon vanilla extract

1 teaspoon lemon juice

Preparation

In a large mixing bowl, add gluten-free flour and salt. Mix until well-combined. Cut your vegetable shortening into 1/2 inch cubes, and using a fork or pastry blender, chop into flour until it forms a grain-like consistency.

Next, beat your egg with 1 tablespoon of the cold, ice water. Pour this over the flour mixture and combine until mixture begins to join. Add more ice water as needed until the dough can hold together when firmly pressed (grab a pinch of dough and roll it into a ball, squeeze this, and if it holds together without crumbling it's good to go!).

Place the dough into the refrigerator to chill for around an hour.

Once your dough is chilled, bring it out and place it onto a well-floured working surface. Form it into a rough ball, and then cut in half.

Set aside one of the halves and save for later. Take the other and, using a rolling pin, begin to roll out the dough until it forms a roughly 10x10 circle, or is about 2 1/2 inches wider than a pie plate.

Preheat the oven to 425° F. In a large bowl, combine pumpkin, eggs, monk fruit sweetener, and coconut cream. Mix thoroughly until combined, add in remaining ingredients, and stir until fully incorporated. Place your pie crust in a ten inch oven-safe pie dish and pour in the filling. Bake at 425° F for 15 minutes, then reduce the heat to 350° F, and allow the pie to continue baking an additional 30-40 minutes, or until a knife inserted into the middle of the pie comes out clean. Remove from the oven and cool for at least one hour (personally I like my pumpkin pie nice and cold so I recommend letting it sit overnight).

Now for the delicious coco-whip topping! Chill your can of coconut milk in the refrigerator overnight, or at least six hours. Once chilled, carefully remove the can.

Scoop out the coconut cream solids only into a large chilled stainless steel bowl, set aside the liquid.

Add in the maple syrup, vanilla, and lemon juice, and using a hand mixer, beat until the cream begins to form soft peaks. That's it, it's ready to serve along with the pumpkin pie. Enjoy!

Serving

After your pie has thoroughly cooled, slice that baby up into eighths, and dole it out. Serve it topped with a hefty dollop of the coco-whip and a sprinkle of cinnamon. All pies are best when shared, so find a few fellow psychonauts and tuck in to a fantastic treat!

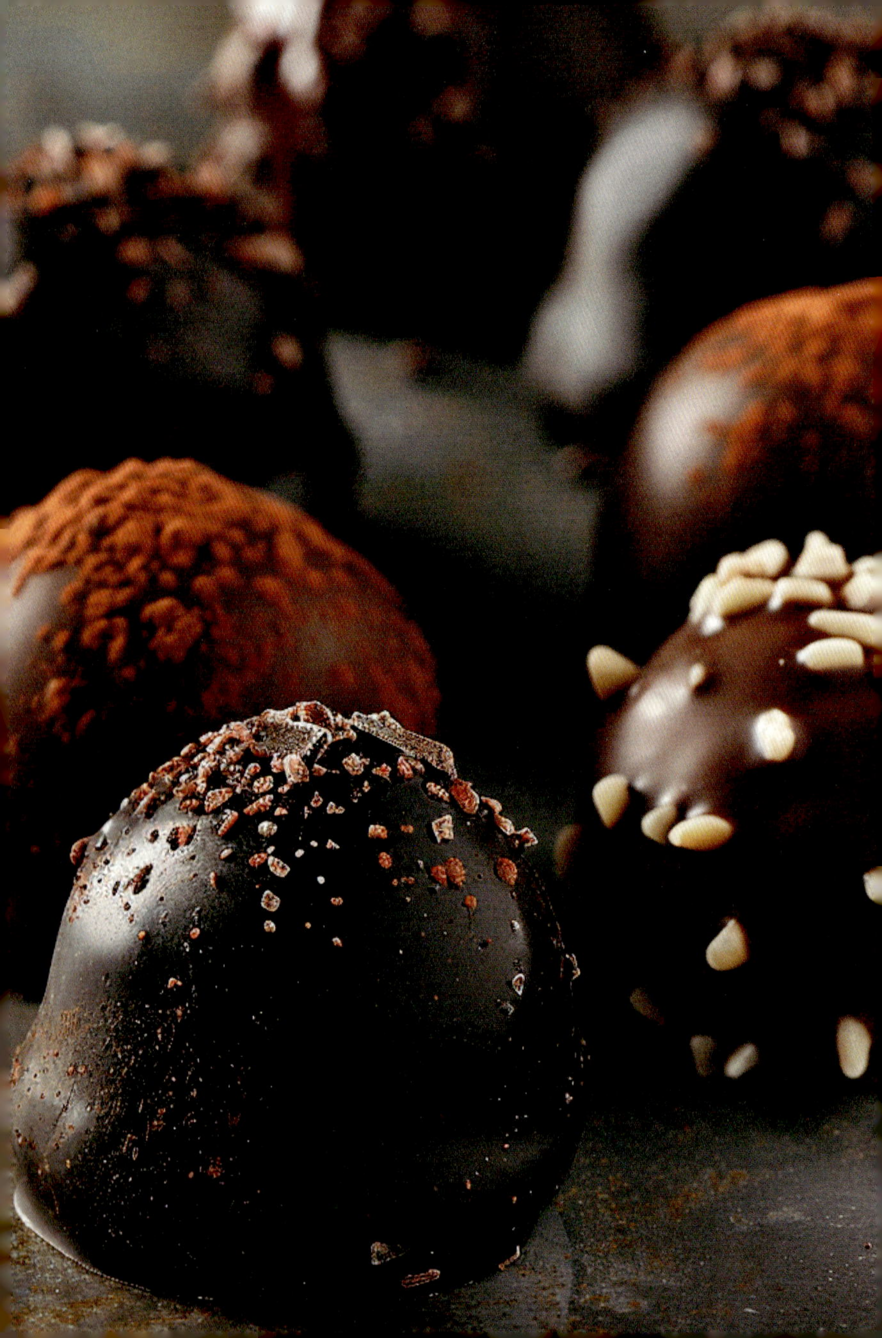

Fantastically Fudgy Fungi Truffles

These fudge-tastic treats are an adapted version of my grandmother's double-fudge chocolate truffles (less sweet and more psychedelic). The 88% dark chocolate shell coats a deliciously decadent fudge center that is complemented by just a hint of earthy mushroom goodness. Make yourself a dozen (the recipe yields 22) and share the rest with your closest chocoholics!

Yield

22 servings

Dose

0.5 grams per serving

Ingredients

1 3/4 cup 88% dark chocolate, roughly chopped (divide out the 3/4 cup)

3/4 cup coconut cream solids (discard the liquid or save for later)

3 tablespoons ghee or coconut oil

4 tablespoons monk fruit sweetener

1/4 tablespoon bourbon vanilla extract

11 ml Mushroom Elixir

Cake pop sticks or toothpicks

Preparation

In a heat-safe bowl, place 1 cup of roughly chopped dark chocolate and set aside. Using a medium saucepan over low heat, pour in the coconut cream, ghee or coconut oil, and sweetener. Stir constantly until the sweetener and ghee/oil have thoroughly mixed with the coconut cream. Take the hot coconut cream mixture and pour this over your chocolate. Stir with a spatula, or whisk, until smooth and totally incorporated (look for a silky-smooth surface). Last, add in the vanilla and Mushroom Elixir, stirring until completely mixed. Place the completed ganache in the refrigerator to cool overnight. Grab yourself a cup of tea, or one of those nifty little smoothies from earlier, and relax for the night!

Shaping

Good morning! I hope you slept well. Now, let's get this last part knocked out and eat some chocolate.

Take up a baking pan and cover it with a piece of wax or parchment paper. Remove the ganache from the refrigerator and begin scooping out the chocolate—using either a small spoon or a melon baller. Continue until the bowl is empty. If your truffles start to get too warm to handle, you can place them in the refrigerator or freezer for a few minutes to firm back up. Next, take the last 3/4 cup of chocolate and place it in a microwave-safe bowl. Begin heating it in 30 second intervals, stirring between until smooth and fully melted.

Using your cake pop sticks or toothpicks, place one in each truffle and then use it to dip the truffles into the melted chocolate. Coating lightly. Keep at it until all the truffles are coated. If you're feeling fancy, garnish them with nuts or cocoa powder. Place them back into the refrigerator and chill until ready to serve.

Serving

This part is complex so pay close attention. Take a truffle off the pan, and pop that little beauty in your mouth. Enjoy with friends, or on your own!

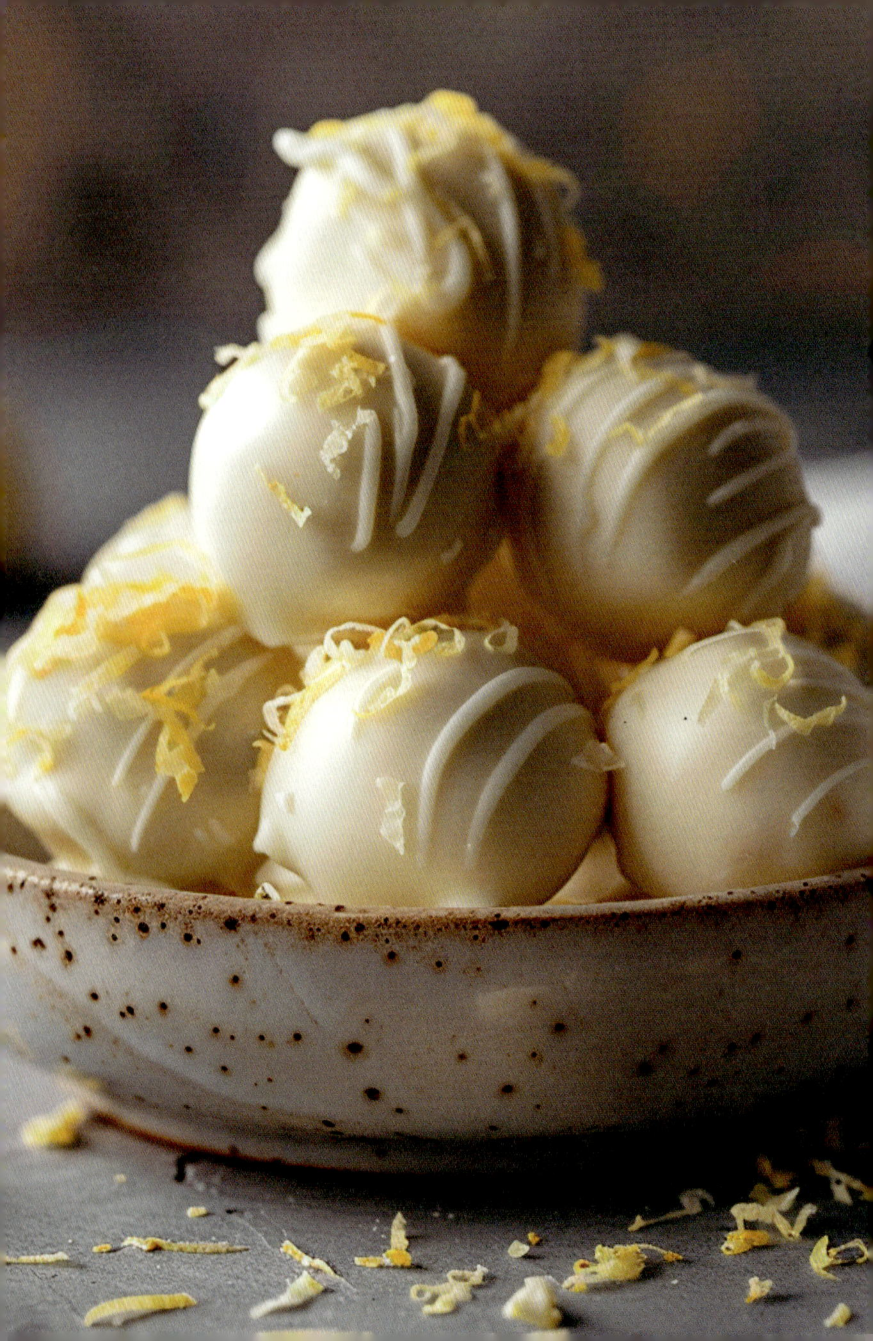

Less Stress Lemon Lime Truffles

The inspiration for these lemony treats came from my grandmother's excellent, but very complex, lemon bar recipe. However, these truffles are light and refreshingly citrusy, and don't take much effort or time. I like to use finely chopped mushrooms soaked in the juice of half a lime and half a lemon, and then strain. With around 50 mg of psilocin (extracted from the fun-guys using a version of the lemon tek from earlier) per truffle, these little guys will open your inner eye without also sending you to Pluto (unless you eat around 6). Enjoy them fresh from the fridge with a cup of warm tea and some cosmically awesome companions.

Yield

22 servings

Dose

0.5 grams per serving

Ingredients

1 1/4 cup cocoa butter pieces

1/2 cup coconut cream solids

4 tablespoons monk fruit sweetener

1/2 lime & 1/2 lemon juiced

Zest of 1 lime (can be omitted)

11 grams finely chopped fun-guys

Topping Options

1/4 cup coconut shredded with 1/2 tablespoon lemon zest

Cocoa powder

Powdered monk fruit sweetener

Preparation

First gather and roughly chop about 11 grams of dried fun-guys. Once chopped, add them to a small bowl and juice half a lemon and half a lime into the bowl. Let this sit for 15-20 minutes, then strain. Using a whisk, mix in the 4 tablespoons of sweetener until fully dissolved. Set your citrus/mushroom juice in the fridge until ready to use.

In a large microwave-safe bowl, combine cocoa butter pieces with the coconut cream solids. Microwave in 30 second intervals, stirring gently and folding in between intervals. Continue until the cocoa butter is completely combined and smooth (yay, no stove top needed!). Remove the bowl of citrus juice blend from the refrigerator, strain out the mushroom material using a fine mesh strainer or cheesecloth, and then slowly pour it into the cocoa butter mix—stirring until thoroughly incorporated. Lastly, zest one lime and mix into your ganache until well distributed. Place your ganache in the refrigerator to chill overnight. At this point, I recommend making some of our Mushroom Toddy's and settling in for a relaxing day or evening.

Welcome back! I swear, you're just the best! Now, get that big, old bowl of ganache out of the fridge and ready your scooping tool of choice. Using either a spoon or melon baller, begin scooping out ganache onto a pan covered with parchment paper. Do this until the bowl is empty. Once done, top the truffles with your favorite toppings—I like to roll them in a mix of cocoa powder and shredded coconut. Put them back in the refrigerator until it's time to serve.

Serving

Grab a few and share with friends. Pairs nicely with Cubensis Coffee or Lavender Mint Tea. These things are perfect for group paint-and-chill sessions or sharing around a campfire!

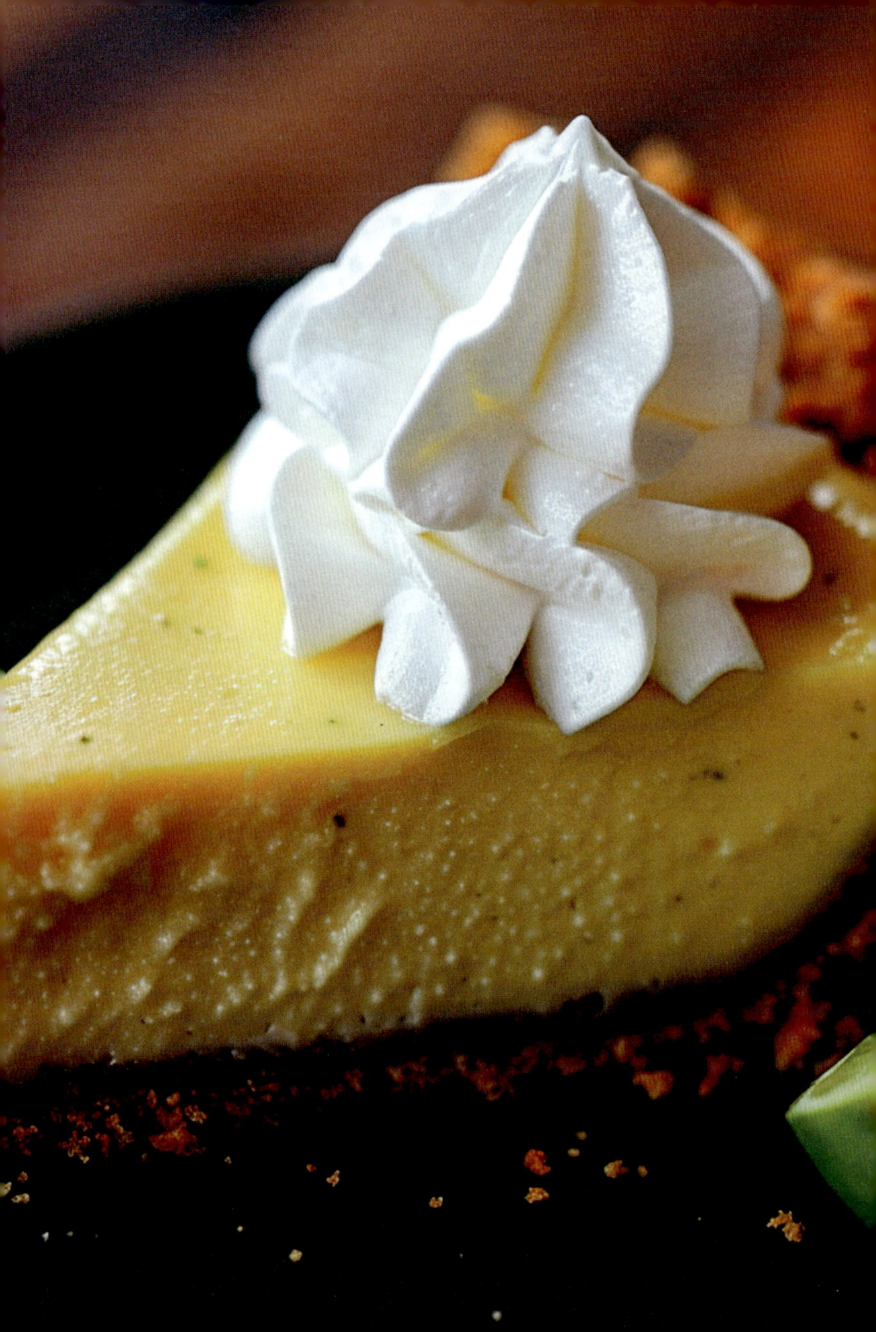

Key Lime and Fun-guy Pie

Like so many of my recipes, this one can only be attributed to my grandmother, whose kitchen wizardry is without compare. My modifications to it make the pie a little lighter on the calories, and free from dairy and added sugars. I have also included a wonderfully flaky recipe for gluten-free pie crust. If you'd prefer the easy route, I find that Trader Joe's and Kroger both offer an excellent frozen pie crust (for those of us looking to save a little time). The flavors from the coconut cream base blend very well with the sharp, brightly acidic Key lime and lemon juice. As far as dosing goes, each slice has just enough punch to have you feeling like you're on Cloud Nine, but is still navigable and shouldn't interfere with your day. Enjoy it on a hot and sunny afternoon or after a good meal (for breakfast is fine too)!

Yield

8 servings

Dose

0.5 grams per serving

Ingredients

1 ten inch gluten-free crust (see page 139)

Filling

1 can coconut cream solids

⅛ teaspoon salt

1/4 cup Key lime juice

⅛ cup lemon juice

1/4 cup monk fruit sweetener

2 large eggs + 1 yolk

Zest of 2 limes

8 ml Mushroom Elixir

Preparation

Preheat your oven to 425° F.

Place one ten inch crust into a 10x10 pie pan, or oven-safe pie dish. Using a fork, prick the bottom of the crust about 50 times (this will keep the crust from blistering or rising during pre-baking). Bake for 10-12 minutes, then set aside to cool.

Lower your oven to 325° F.

Fillin'

In a medium saucepan, combine your lemon juice, salt, and coconut cream over medium heat—stirring occasionally. Beat your two eggs and the one yolk together. Using a whisk, slowly begin to incorporate your eggs with the coconut cream and citrus juice. Stir this continuously. Next, add in the 1/4 cup of sweetener and lime zest. Once thoroughly combined, cook your custard until the mixture starts becoming slightly thick and viscous. Place this to the side to cool for 15 minutes before mixing in the 8 ml of Mushroom Elixir.

Bringing it all together

Once you have finished cooking your custard, slowly pour it into the pre-baked pie crust. Place this in the oven to bake for 35-40 minutes, or until a butter knife inserted into the middle of the pie comes out clean. After baking, allow the pie to cool on a pie rack for at least four hours then move it into the refrigerator overnight.

Serving

I really like this served up with a corkscrew of fresh lime and a big dollop of our homemade coco-whip (the creaminess really helps counter balance the tang of the pie). Slice it up into eighths and dole it out to your eagerly awaiting friends. This pairs well with the Cold Brew version of Cubensis Coffee!

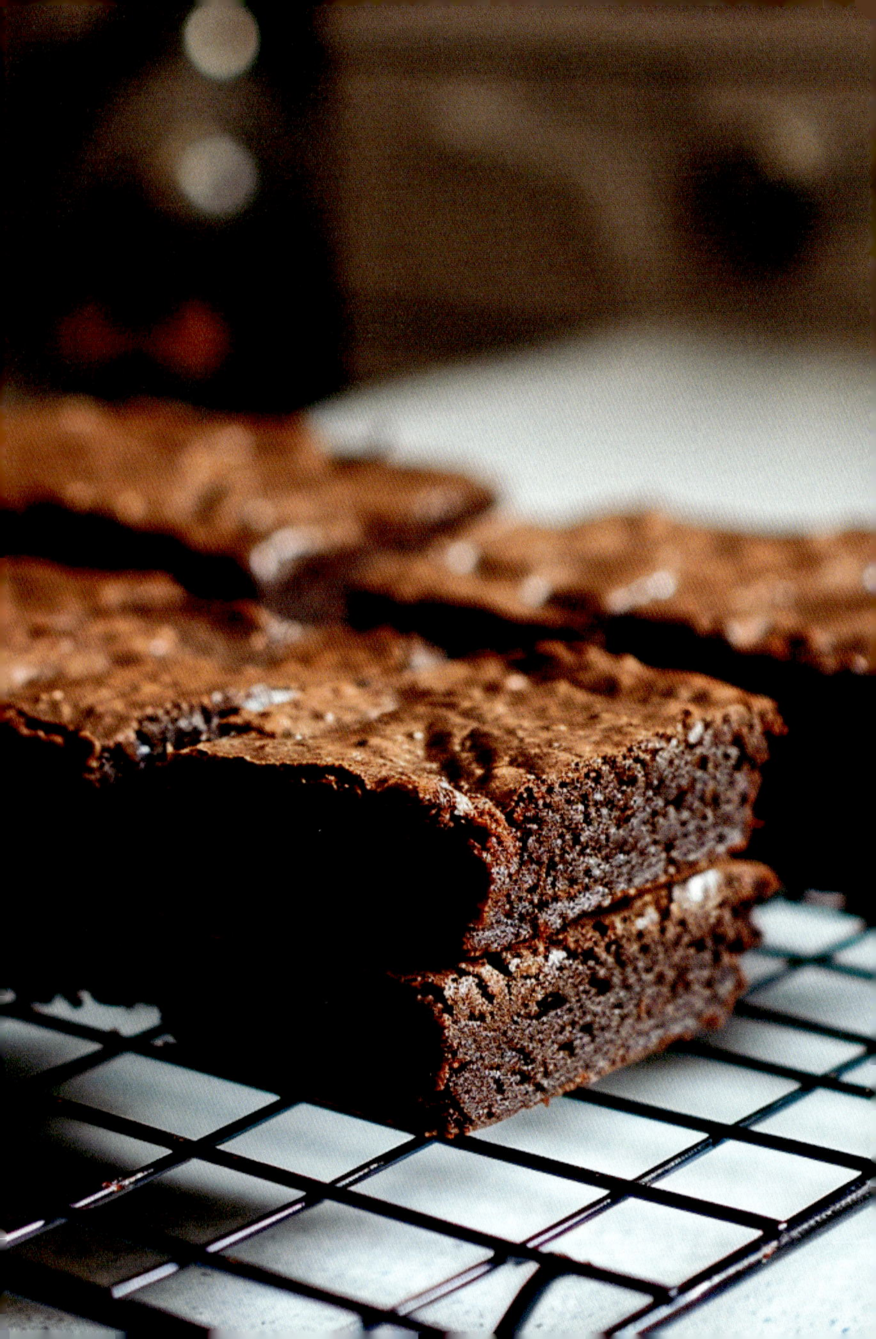

Celestial Psilocybin Avocado Brownies

This is a creation via my cousin, Steve (she's a cosmically amazing unicorn of a person). The brownies are decadently chocolatey, without being too heavy on the calories. Devoid of added sugar, as well as dairy- and gluten-free, these little treats are ready to impress. It's also a super simple and quick recipe, which makes it perfect for putting together before an evening kickback with your crew.

Yield

16 servings

Dose

0.5 grams per serving

Ingredients

4 oz 88% dark chocolate 2 tablespoons extra-virgin olive oil

2 large ripe avocados, peeled and thoroughly mashed

2 eggs, beaten

1/4 cup monk fruit sweetener

3 drops liquid liquid sugar substitute

3/4 cup coconut milk

1 1/2 cup gluten-free all-purpose flour (I like Arrowhead for its consistency)

1/4 + 1/4 cup unsweetened dark cocoa powder, divided

1 1/2 teaspoon vanilla bourbon extract

8 grams powdered funguys

Preparation

Preheat the oven to 375° F. Roughly chop your chocolate, and using a small, microwave-safe bowl heat in 30 second intervals until the chocolate is fully melted—stir between intervals. In a large mixing bowl, combine all dry ingredients, including the powdered fungi. Using a fork or spatula, mix this until everything is completely combined and distributed. Next, add the vanilla, liquid sugar substitute, eggs, and oil. Stir until mixed through and then add in your melted chocolate. Stir again until combined.

Pour the mix into a prepared 10x10 baking dish and let it bake for 25 minutes, or until a butter knife comes out of the center clean. Let cool for at least 20 minutes.

Serving

Using your remaining 1/4 cup of cocoa powder, dust the brownies. Slice off a few pieces and pair it with our Star-Side Fungiccinos and a few best friends for an incredible journey into cosmic insight and creativity. It's also pretty good with some fresh coco-whip or just on its own. Remember to keep an eye on your dosing and have a great time!

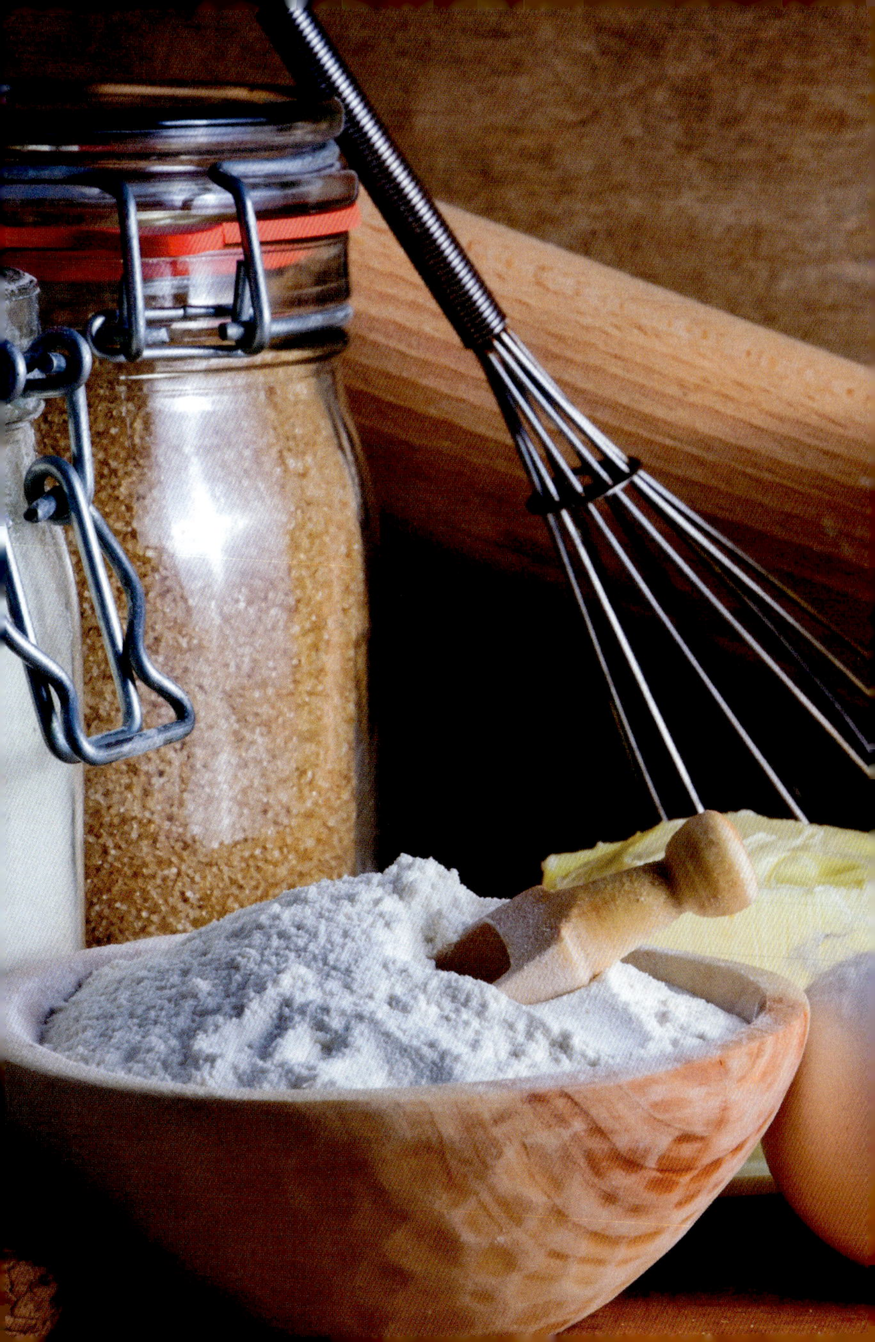

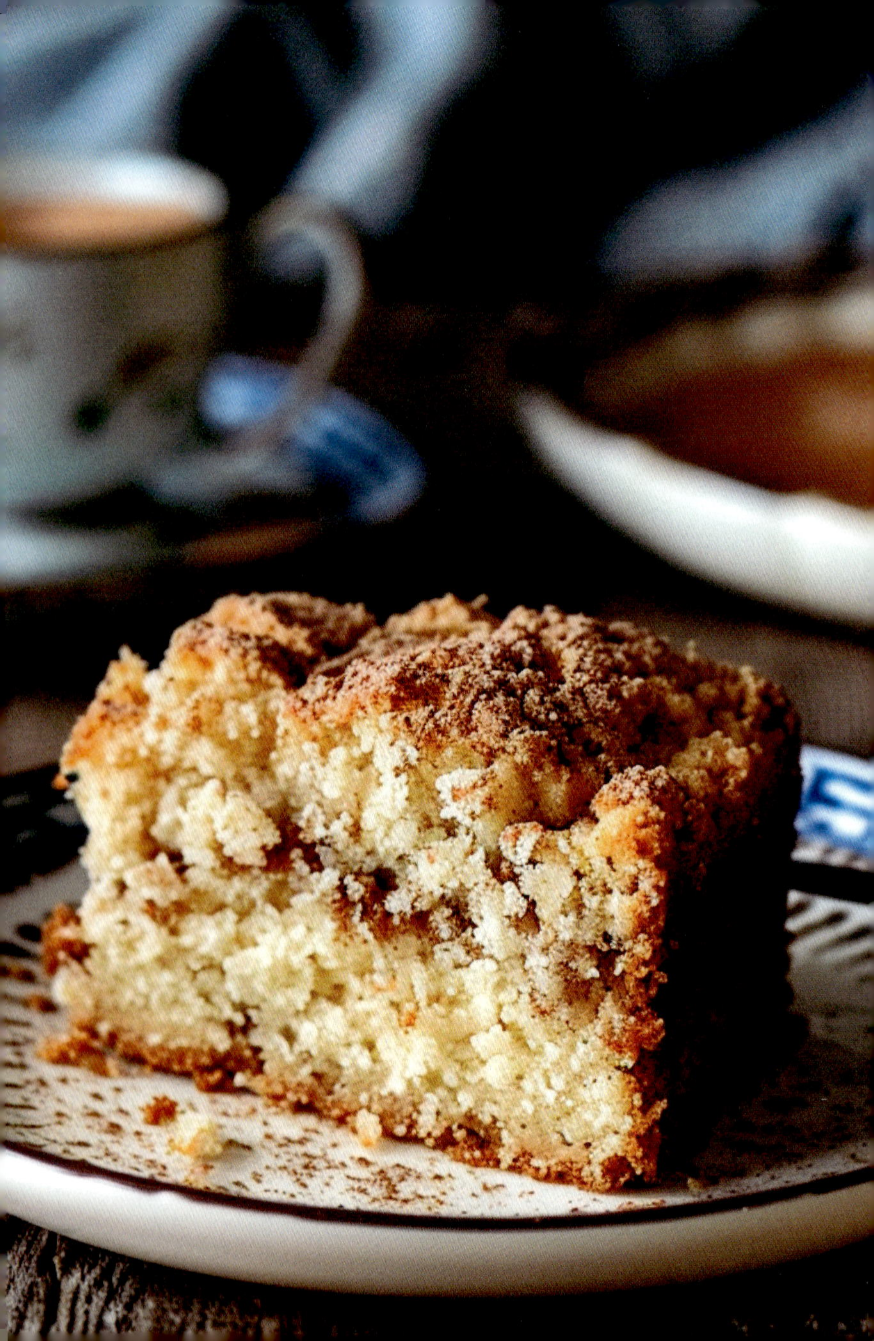

Cubensis Coffee Cake

This recipe was given to us by our friend and amazing artist, Snowflake. It is a wonderfully light treat that pairs with any of our coffee recipes. We like to use the left-over grinds from the Cubensis Coffee (see page 121), which fully uses the mushroom and eliminates some waste (every little bit left out of the rubbish helps). My only alterations are the replacement of the dairy, sugar, and substitution of gluten-free flour to make this a truly guilt-free (and celiac friendly) treat that's still delicious and approachable.

Yield

8 servings

Dose

< 0.5 grams per serving

Ingredients

1 3/4 cup gluten-free all-purpose flour

3/4 teaspoon baking soda

3/4 teaspoon baking powder

3/4 teaspoon cinnamon

1/2 teaspoon salt

1/4 teaspoon nutmeg

1/2 cup strong brewed coffee

1 tablespoon Cubensis Coffee grinds, dried out and very finely powdered (just use regular to control the dosing)

1/3 cup coconut cream solids

1 cup ghee or coconut oil (room temp)

3/4 cup monk fruit sweetener (or similar granulated sugar replacement)

2 eggs

1 teaspoon bourbon vanilla

Preparation

Preheat Oven to 350° F.

In a large mixing bowl, begin by combining your dry ingredients—whisk them until fully incorporated (including the dried and powdered coffee grinds). In a small saucepan over very low heat, begin to mix the coconut cream and coffee. Do not allow it to come to a simmer, simply warm and melt the coconut cream solids, and incorporate that with the coffee. Once mixed, pour your cream over the dry ingredients and whisk until smooth and combined (make sure you go all the way to the bottom of the bowl to break up any leftover dry ingredients).

In a separate bowl, whisk together the room temperature ghee and sweetener until light and fluffy (the fluffier the better). Adding one at a time, begin to whisk in your eggs—mix until thoroughly combined and smooth. Next, add the vanilla and beat until soft peaks begin to form.

Take the eggs and butter mixture and begin folding it into the batter. Do this slowly until the batter is smooth and completely joined (the key here is to gently fold batter so it stays nice and fluffed).

Put the batter into a 9x9 baking dish and let it bake for about 45 minutes, or until a butter knife comes out clean when inserted into the middle. Allow to cool for at least 30 minutes before serving.

Serving

Serve the coffee cake alongside a cup of Cubensis Coffee, or any of our other coffee drinks. It is also very nice with our Mushroom Toddy recipe. As always, I like mine topped off with a little fresh coco-whip, but others insist that it's best as is (like with so many other things in life, there is no wrong answer). Share this with a few fellow wanderers of life and enjoy!

Safety Note: Since we are using brewed coffee grinds, the dosage will be more difficult to determine so please USE CAUTION when enjoying with other food or drink from this book.

FUNGI-FORWARD FARE

CHAPTER EIGHT

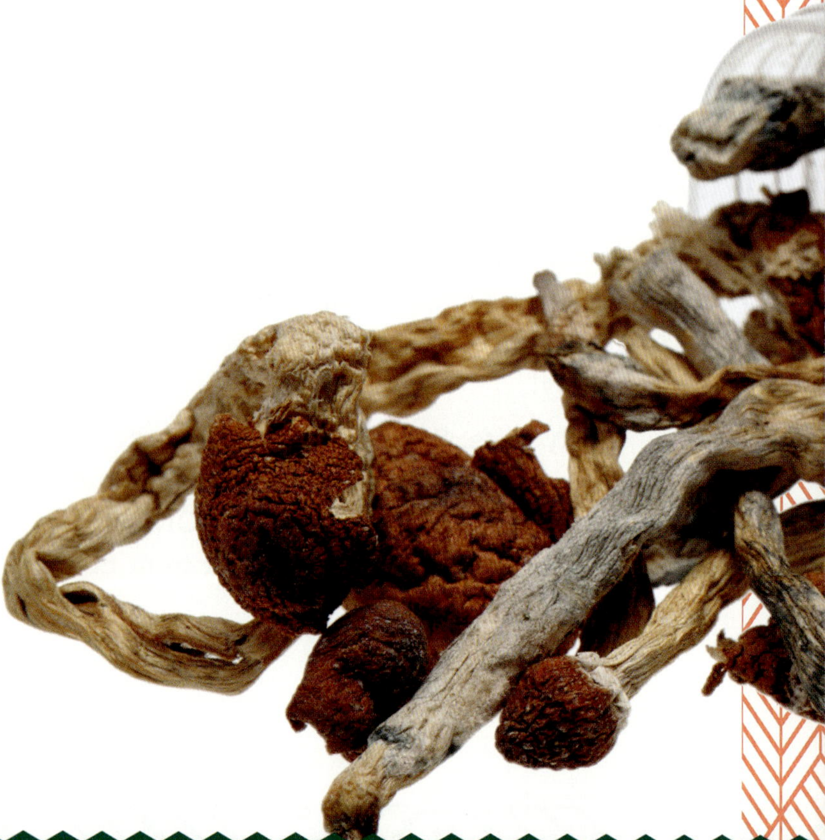

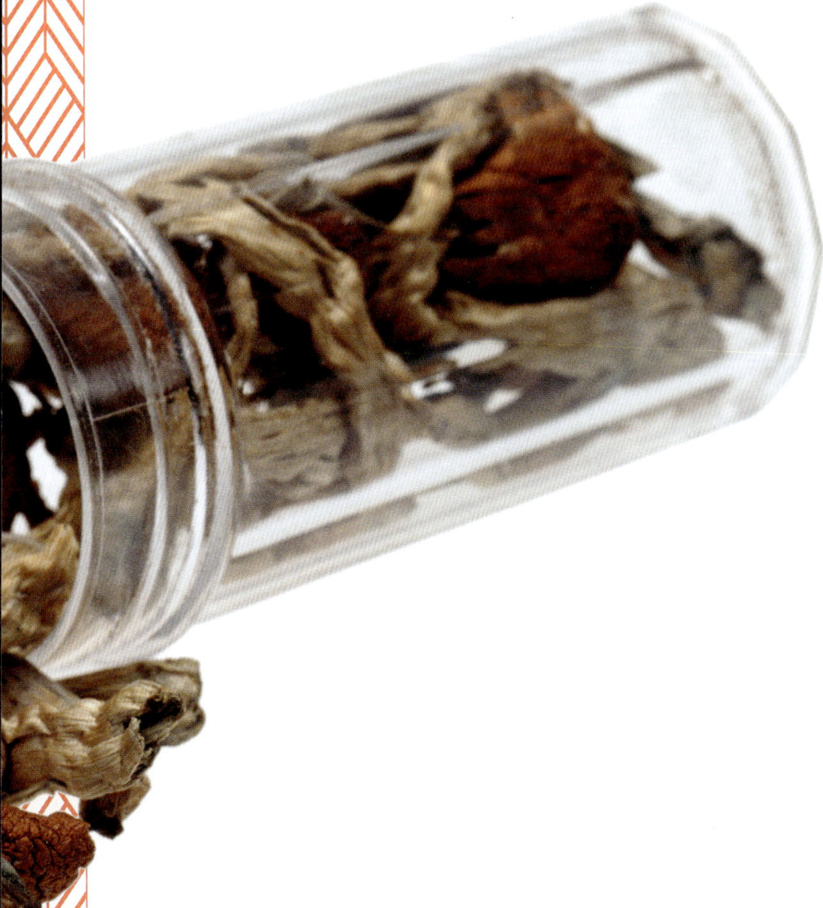

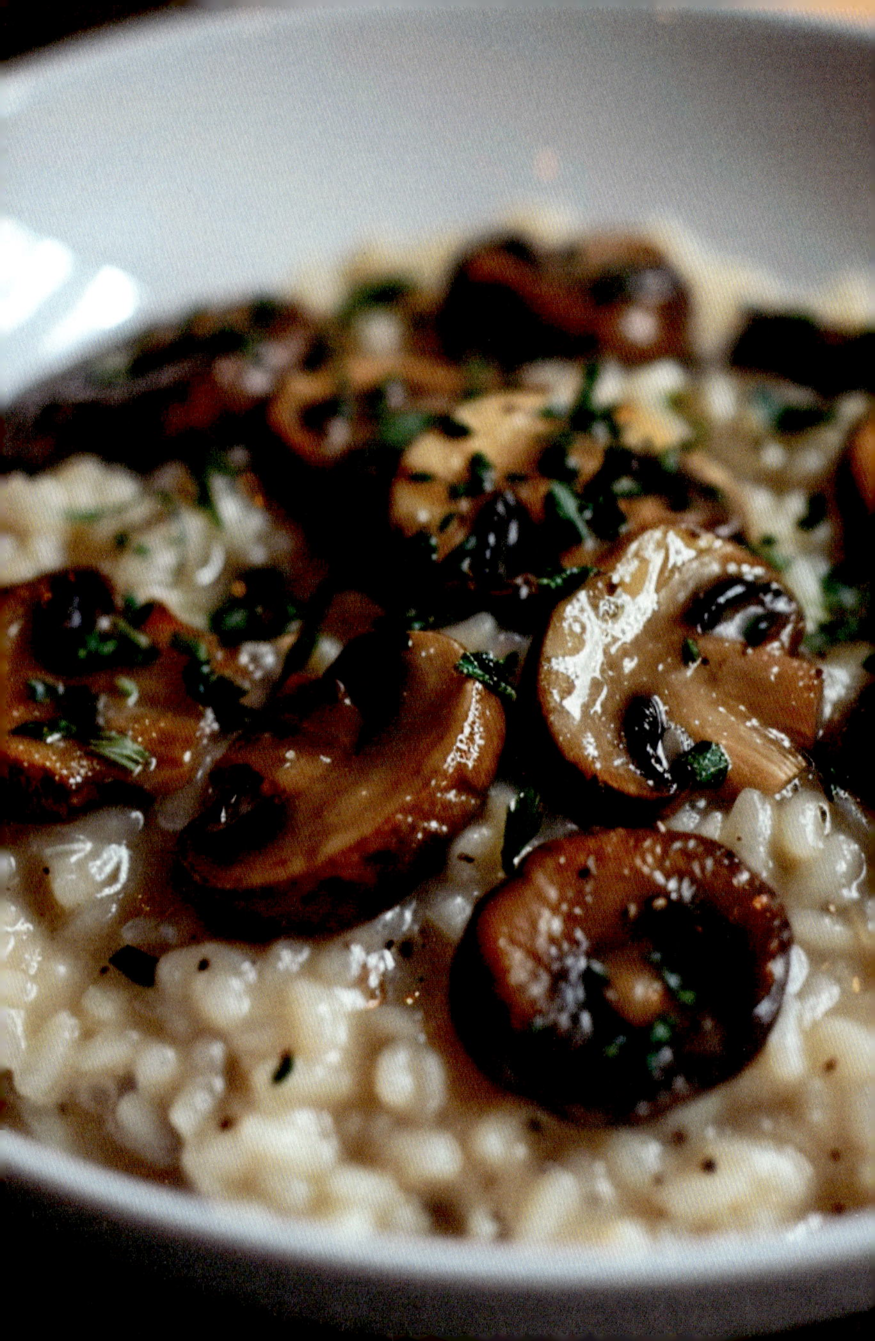

Radical Risotto with Freshies and Shiitakes

My personal take on an old mushroom risotto recipe I found in a cookbook years ago; I've taken out the dairy and replaced it with a combination of vegan cheese and dietary yeast (which is surprisingly good). It is best when prepared with Freshies, but if those are hard to come by you can use reconstituted dry Magic Mushrooms. Paired with the shiitakes, this makes for a delicious and enlightening meal. Be sure to keep an eye on your serving size, this risotto is so good it may be hard to resist overeating (and thus over-dosing). As always, use common sense and safe practices. Enjoy my friends!

Yield

8 servings

Dose

0.5 per serving

Ingredients

8 oz stemmed shiitake mushrooms

40 grams fresh psilocybin (if using reconstituted mushrooms start with 4 grams dried and roughly chopped)

2 tablespoons extra-virgin olive oil

2 1/2 tablespoons ghee

1 small, sweet onion, diced (I like Vidalia if you can get them)

2 cloves garlic (chiffonade)

2 tablespoons extra-virgin olive oil

1 cup long grain wild rice

1/3 cup dry white wine (plus some more for sipping, cooking can be thirsty work)

2 1/2 cups chicken or vegetable stock

3/4 cups Thrive Parmesan Alternative

1 tablespoon nutritional yeast

Salt and pepper to taste

Preparation

Before we get started, note that the key to cooking with fresh Magic Mushrooms is low, slow heat. Psilocybin breaks down in high temperatures, so we want to avoid rapidly cooking the fruits. So, let's get to it!

Start off by cleaning both sets of mushrooms, if at all possible just brush them off and avoid washing. Roughly slice the shiitake and the Freshies (if you have smaller Freshies just slice them lengthwise down the middle).

In a medium saucepan, heat 2 tablespoons of oil and 2 tablespoons of ghee on medium heat. Set the rest of the ghee aside for later. Add in the shiitakes *only*, and sauté until lightly browned and tender, salt and pepper them slightly, and allow to cook for another minute or so. Next, reduce the heat to low and add in the Freshies (or rehydrated dried mushrooms). Allow the fungi to cook until they are all tender. Remove from heat and set aside.

Using a medium-large saucepan, melt the remaining ghee and olive oil together. Throw in the diced onion and cook until slightly caramelized, then add garlic and heat until fragrant. Add in the wild rice and cook until just barely toasted.

Quickly add your white wine, stirring all the while to deglaze the pan. Next, pour in 1/4 cup of your stock of choice (stir this constantly, adding more stock, 1/4 cup at a time, until fully absorbed by the rice).

Cook your rice until tender, this takes about 25 minutes. Remove from heat and add in your vegan cheese and dietary yeast. Mix, then salt and pepper to taste. Lastly, add in the mushrooms and stir it all together. Let cool for around seven minutes or so.

Serving

Plate this wonderfully warming dish with a sprinkle of vegan parmesan and fresh chopped rosemary, with a little parsley, to add a nice herbal touch. Serve alongside a fresh spring salad and a nice earthy Nebbiolo or Pinot Noir, and, of course, don't forget to bring some pals for this soul-feeding feast!

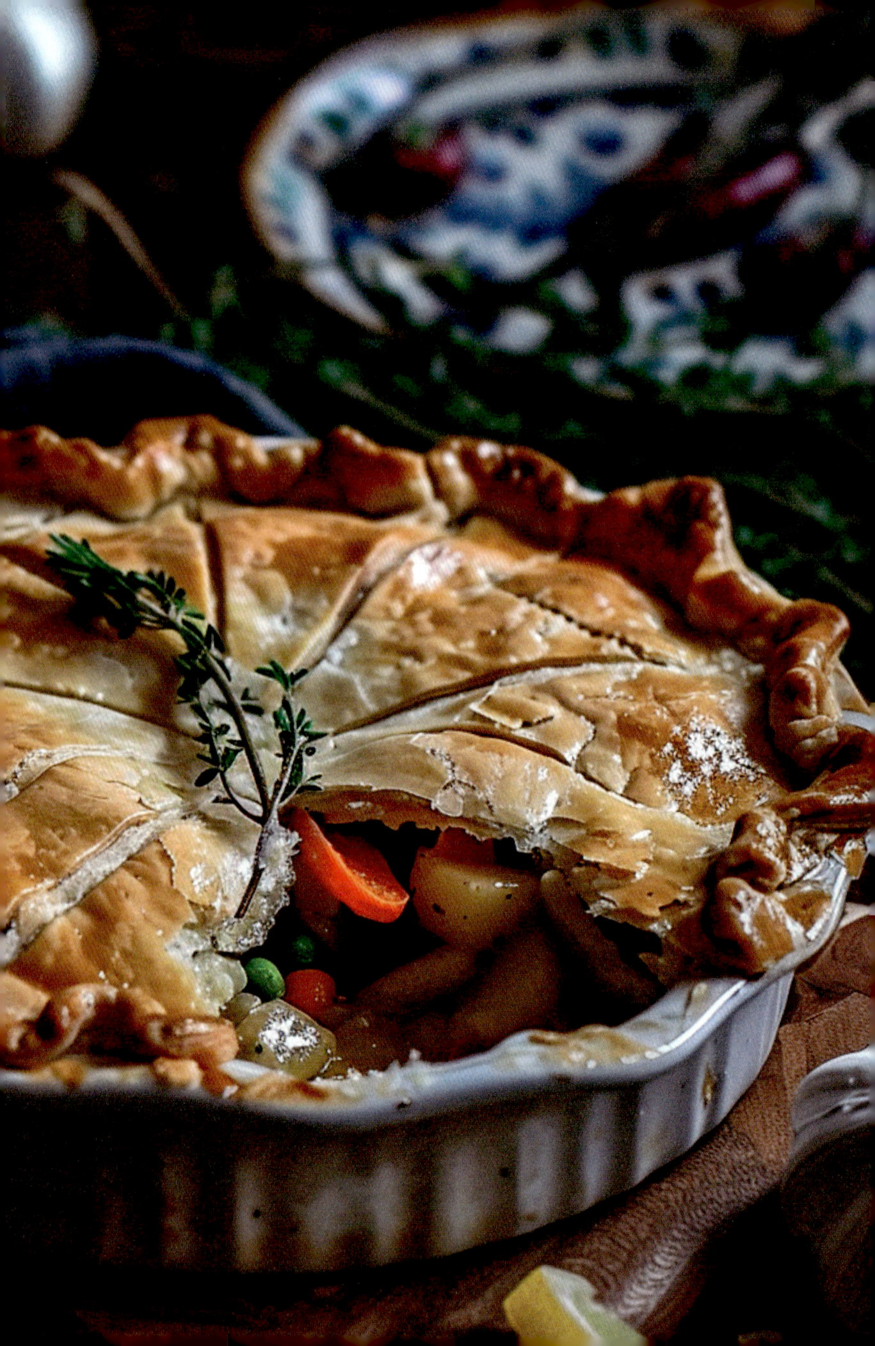

Magically Mushroomed Pot Pie

Meat-free and majestic is the best way to describe this vegetarian delight. We partnered with a close friend, and self-professed pot pie fanatic, to bring you a dish that's sure to warm your belly and your soul. Our team combined delicious oyster mushrooms, with neurogenesis fueling Lion's Mane, and, of course, *Psilocybe cubensis* to create this food phenomenon. Using our Gluten-Free Pie crust (page 139), ensures that this alluringly delicious pie is approachable for all.

SAFETY NOTE: The dosing in this one is a little heavier than some of our other recipes so please approach it with care (and of course feel free to lower it as needed, or raise it for that matter).

Yield

8 servings

Dose

1.5 grams per serving

Ingredients

2 tablespoons extra-virgin olive oil

18 oz fresh oyster mushrooms, chopped

6 oz fresh lion's mane mushrooms, chopped

12 grams powdered Magic Mushrooms

6 carrots, diced

2 cups of russet potatoes, diced

4 celery stalks, diced

1 medium onion, roughly chopped

3/4 teaspoon thyme

1/3 cup Arrowhead Gluten-Free All-Purpose Flour

1 1/2 cups vegetable stock

1 cup frozen peas

Gluten-free pie crust (halved and rolled into 10x10 sheets)

Salt and pepper

Preparation

Preheat the oven to 400° F. In a large cast iron skillet, using medium-high heat, pre-heat the olive oil. When that's ready, add in carrots, oyster and lion's mane mushrooms, celery, onions, and potatoes. Stirring occasionally, allow the vegetables to cook until tender, add in the thyme, and then season with salt and pepper. Next, add in the flour, stirring it constantly until cooked. Pour in your broth and frozen peas, bring to a fast simmer until thickened. At this point, take a little taste and add more salt and pepper as needed. Remove from heat and allow to cool for 15 minutes, then stir in your powdered fun-guys (we don't want it to get too hot or they'll lose their potency and be rendered magicless).

Take a 9x9 pie dish and add in one of the rolled crusts. Pour in your pie filling and cover with the second crust. Roll the edges together to seal the pie, and cut three slits across the top to allow it to vent. This will keep your filling from spilling over and making a giant mess.

Place the pie in the oven and bake for around 45 minutes, or until the crust is uniformly golden brown. Let it rest and cool for approximately 20 minutes before serving.

Serving

Slice this gorgeous, savory concoction into eighths and lay it out with a fresh summer salad. It pairs very well with a luscious Merlot. Make sure to invite your closest confidants and tuck in for a hearty and heartening meal!

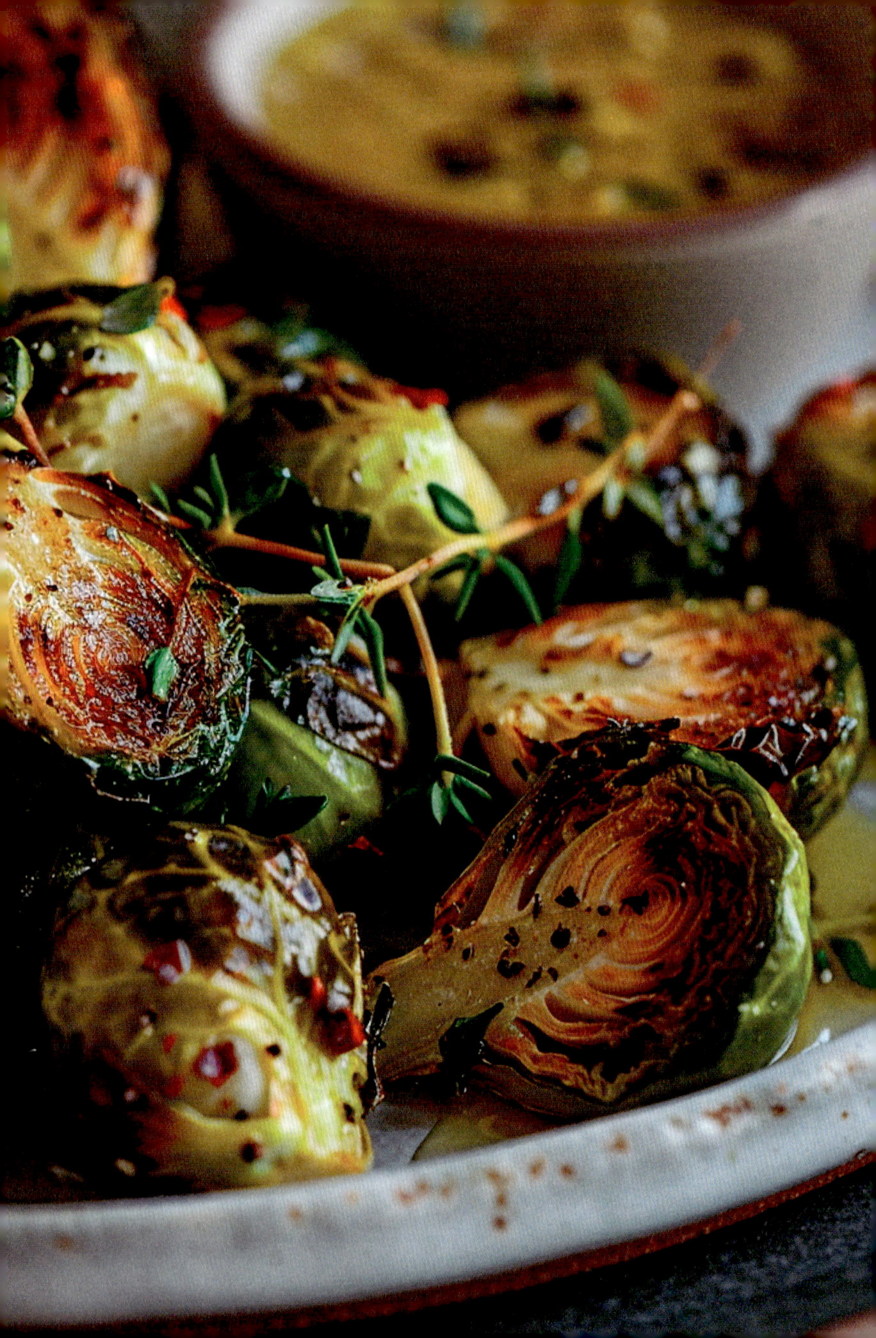

Mushroom Dusted Roast Brussel Sprouts in Mustard Sauce

I whipped this delightful, and nutrient dense, dish up on one of our weekly meat-free days. The Brussels sprouts and roasted baby bella mushrooms are complemented by an amazing Dijon mustard sauce, and, of course, they are dusted with a little psilocybin seasoning blend for some added magic. Served hot or cold, this dish makes a great main, or pair it with our Mushroom Risotto for a frighteningly good feast.

Yield

6 servings

Dose

0.5 grams per serving

Ingredients

1 pound Brussels sprouts, cleaned and halved

1/2 pound baby bellas, whole

1/4 cup extra-virgin olive oil

2 large shallots, diced and divided

2 teaspoons mustard seed

6 strips Sweet Earth vegan bacon

3 grams powdered fun-guys

1/4 cup white wine

1 tablespoon Dijon mustard

Salt and Pepper to taste

Preparation

Begin by preheating your oven to 400° F. Rinse and halve your Brussels sprouts, and gently brush off the baby bellas. In a roasting pan, toss the mushrooms, sprouts, and olive oil with a good amount of salt and pepper. Add in the mustard seed and half of the shallots. Roast the sprouts and bellas in the oven for 25-35 minutes, or until tender and a little crisp.

In a medium pan, fry up the vegan bacon until crisp—remove this from the heat and set it aside. Drizzle a little more olive oil, add the shallots, and cook until translucent. Add in the white wine and Dijon, and using a spatula (or some such implement of cookery) scrape the bottom of the pan to free up all the caramelized goodness. Salt and pepper to taste. Remove from heat and set aside to cool slightly.

Once fully cooked and crispy, remove the Brussels sprouts and baby bella mushrooms from the oven. Crush up the vegan bacon and mix it with the powdered mushrooms into your mustard sauce—stirring to thoroughly combine. Toss this with the Brussels sprouts and baby bellas in the roasting pan.

Serving

This is a tough one. How best to eat these delicious, little veggies and their baby bella buddies? Honestly, just put them in a bowl and enjoy—no need to get complicated. As always, share with friends and enjoy yourselves!

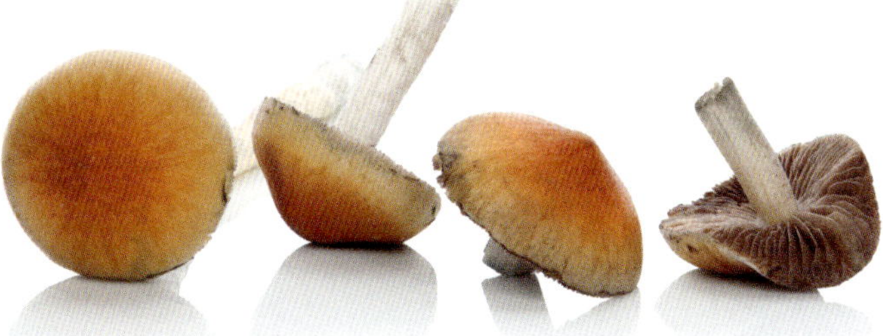

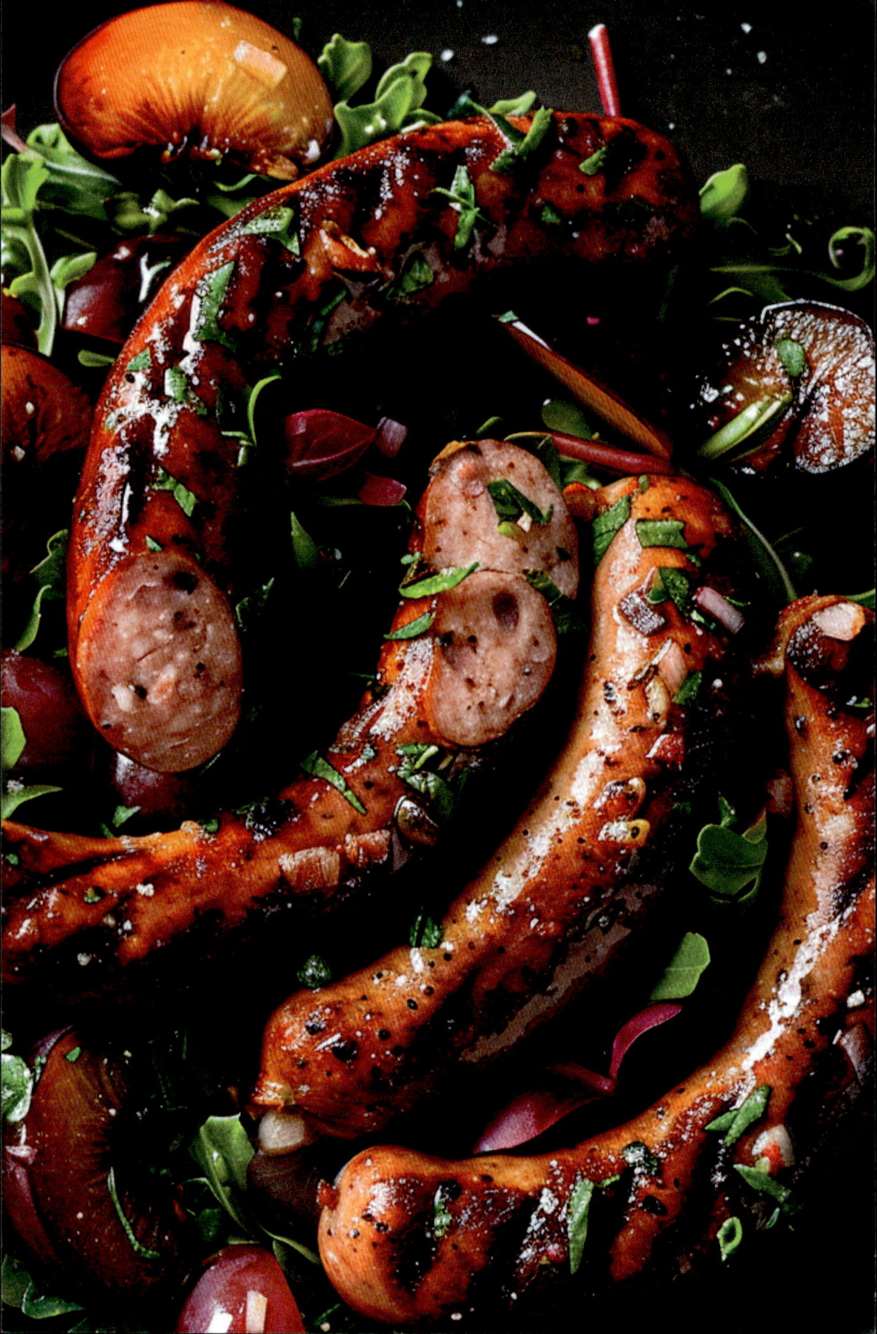

Funky Fungi with Sausage, Plums, and Greens

This is one of our favorite quick and easy dinners to have with friends right before we embark on a solid soul-searching trip. The fresh greens and mustard sauce go very nicely with the warm, spicy sausages and sweet plums. Paired with a nice, crisp glass of cold Riesling, or (if you're wanting to take your trip up a notch) some of our Cool Mint Lime Tea. As with all of our dishes, it's best when enjoyed with some fellow soul searchers and, as always, BE SAFE and enjoy!

Yield

6 servings

Dosage

1 gram per serving (approximately)

Ingredients

6 chicken and rosemary sausages (or whatever kind you like)

1 Vidalia onion, halved and thinly sliced

16 oz fresh greens (I like to use a blend of arugula, baby spinach, and baby kale)

6 fresh plums (stones removed and quartered)

6 grams dried Psilocybe cubensis (reconstituted in vegetable stock)

1/4 cup fresh basil

1/4 cup fresh mint

1/8 cup lemon juice

1 tablespoon Dijon mustard

2 tablespoons balsamic vinegar

1/4 cup extra-virgin olive oil

1/4 cup good white wine

Preparation

First things first, cook your sausages however you like. We grill ours over medium-high heat until they are a nice red/gold brown with defined grill marks. For the onions, sauté them over medium-high heat, with a little oil, until they are translucent and slightly caramelized. Add in the quartered plums and continue to cook until they are warmed through. Once done, pour in the white wine to deglaze the pan—let this simmer until slightly thickened. Remove from heat and set the onions and plums to the side.

While the sausages cook, submerge your dried mushrooms in vegetable stock for approximately 15 minutes or until they are soft and springy. Then whisk together your Dijon mustard, 3 tablespoons of oil, vinegar, and some salt and pepper. Set this to the side (don't forget to check on those sausages). Remove the reconstituted fun-guys from the stock and dice them. Add these, and your lemon juice, to the mustard sauce and whisk it until well-mixed (you can also pour in the stock if you'd like, but it will thin out your sauce).

Once the sausages are fully cooked, let them cool, slice them up, and then toss them together with your onions and plums until they are well-coated in the white wine sauce. Next, toss your greens with the mushroom and mustard sauce (don't be shy with the sauce, get your greens wetter than a summer shower).

Serving

Divide out six portions of greens and pour over sausage, onions, and plums. Top this all off with the fresh basil and mint. You can salt and pepper to taste if you like, but we think this is great as is. Serve it up to your best and brightest friends, then sit back and let the magic kick in!

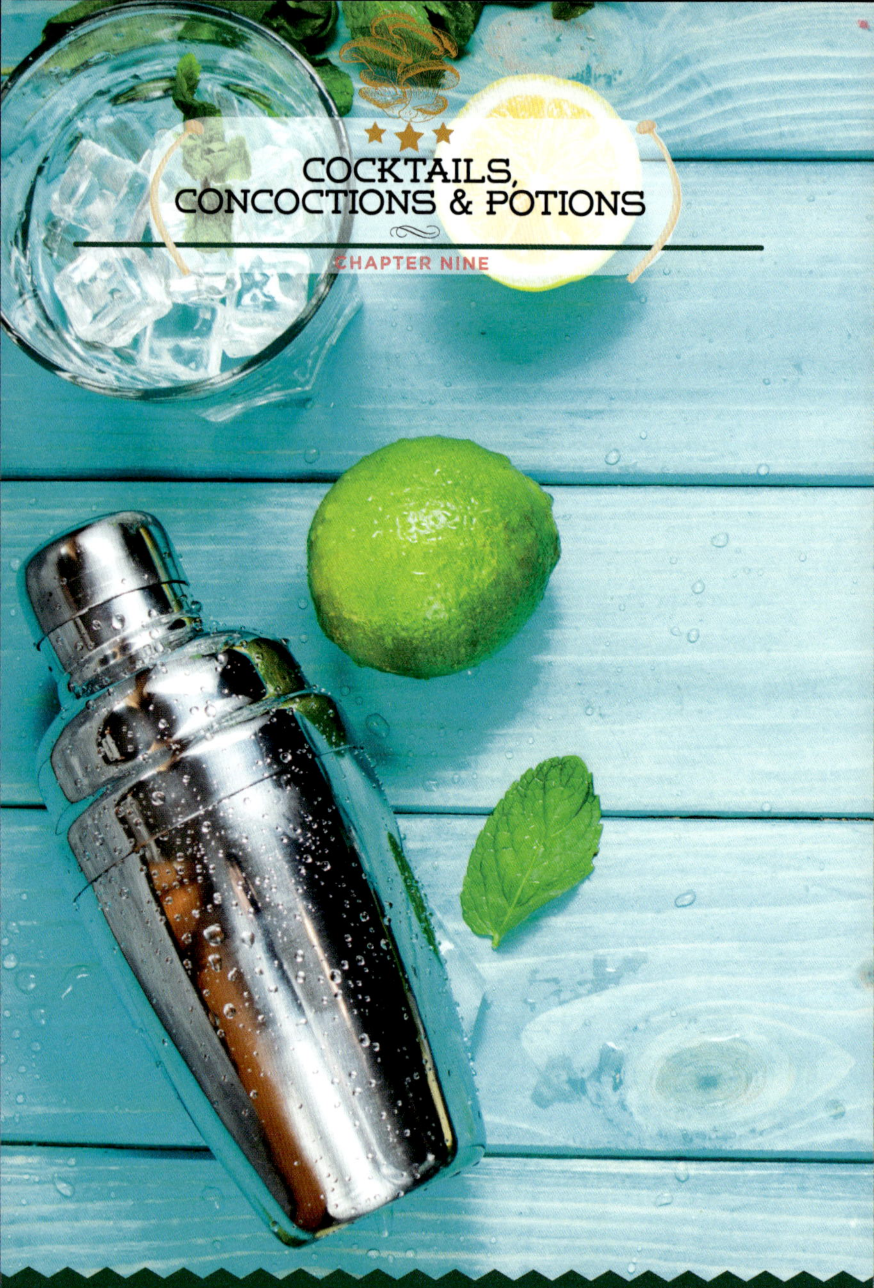

COCKTAILS, CONCOCTIONS & POTIONS

CHAPTER NINE

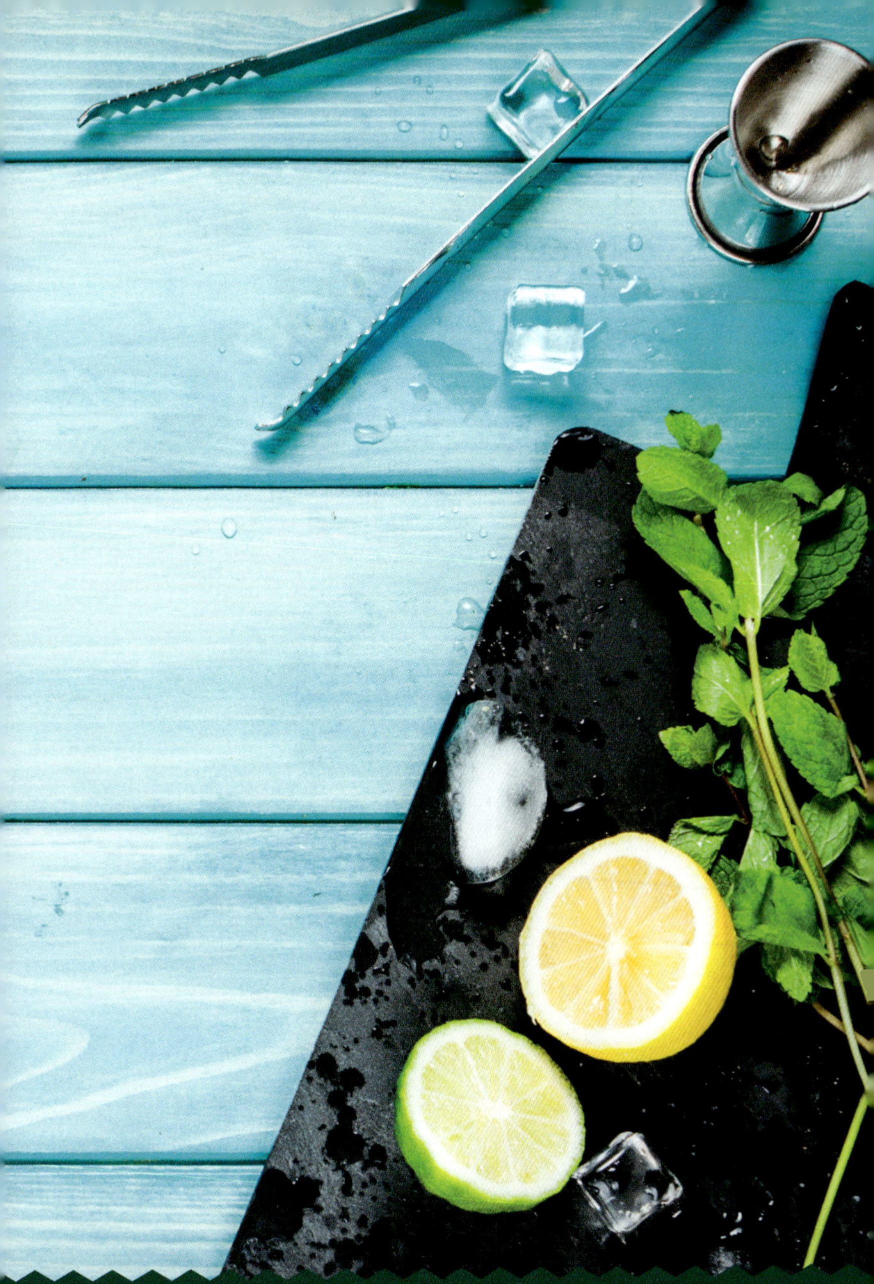

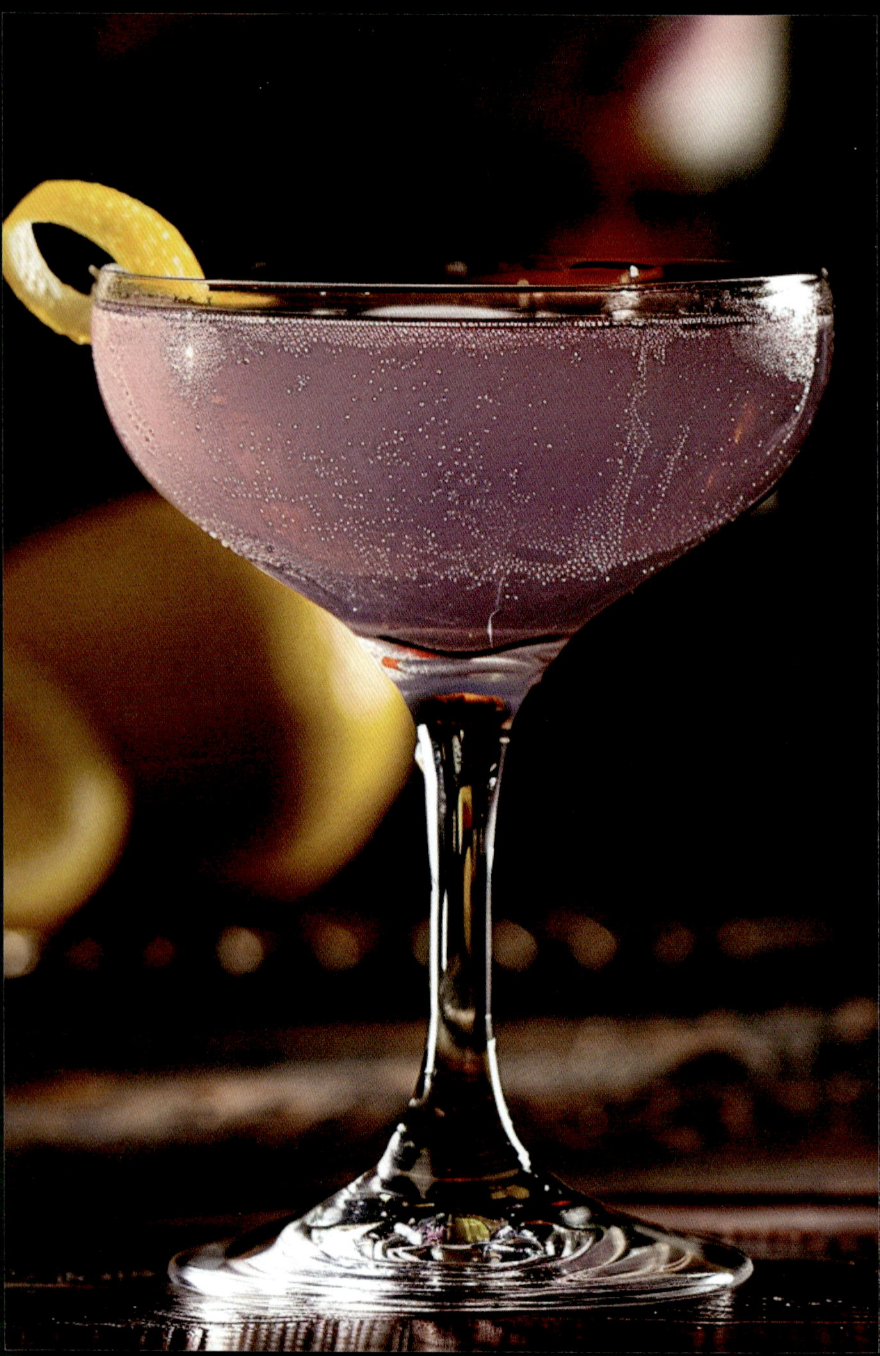

Fairies Blush Cocktail

This lovely refresher is my version of a Maiden's Blush sour, originally invented by the masters at Dead Rabbit Grocery and Grog. I've removed the added sugar from the Raspberry Cordial recipe, and slightly upped the citric acid contents to allow for an easier citric extraction and conversion of psilocin. We've also reduced the alcohol content as much as we could (for safety) while trying to preserve the essential flavors. All in all, you get a deliciously fresh cocktail that doesn't hit hard, but will wake your creative side and ease you into a long evening of introspection and appreciation. Scale this up as needed to share with your chosen few.

Yield

1 serving

Dose

1 gram per serving

Raspberry Cordial

3 oz fresh raspberries

2 cups monk fruit sweetener

2 cups water

1 drop rose extract

1/2 oz Everclear

Cocktail

1 gram dried fun-guys, finely chopped

1 1/4 oz sugar-free raspberry cordial

1/2 oz fresh lime juice

1 1/2 oz Empress 1908 Gin

Preparation

In a blender, purée the raspberries until smooth. Pour the purée into a small mixing bowl and set aside. In a small saucepan, combine sweetener and water over medium heat, do not allow this to come to a boil. When the sugar-free syrup has been reduced, and begins to thicken (you're looking for a slightly viscous fluid, this may take around ten minutes), remove from heat and allow to cool completely. Add the raspberries and stir to combine. Cover and let your mixture cool in the refrigerator overnight. Since you've worked so hard feel free to make some tea and take a break!

Hello again, let's wrap this up. Take a mason jar, or 16 oz bottle, and two coffee filters (the same conical ones we used for the Elixir work well here). Double up and insert the coffee filters into your jar, or bottle, leaving about half an inch sticking out. Fold the edges over and use a rubber band to secure the filters.

Get the raspberry mixture out of the refrigerator and begin to pour it into the filters, allowing time for it to drain before refilling. Gently pat the mixture from time to time. Let this sit until all the liquid has drained into your jar. Add the rose extract and Everclear to the bottle. Shake to mix.

This cordial will store in the refrigerator for up to four weeks.

In a stainless-steel cocktail shaker, combine the fresh lime juice, gin, and finely chopped mushrooms. Let this soak for 15 minutes. Next, add the raspberry cordial, fill with ice, and shake until very well-chilled.

Serving

Strain the cocktail into a wide mouth, or "coupe" style, champagne glass over a single cube of Frozen Blue Juice (see page 101). This beautiful mixer is a wonder to behold. The citric acid from the lemon juice causes the Empress 1908 Gin to transform from its already gorgeous deep blue to an eye-popping shade of lavender. When blended with the raspberry cordial the result is a lovely violet-esque color, hence the name "Fairies Blush." The end product is a not-too-boozy but flavor intense beverage that will add a little color to your cheeks, and a lot of clarity to your mind.

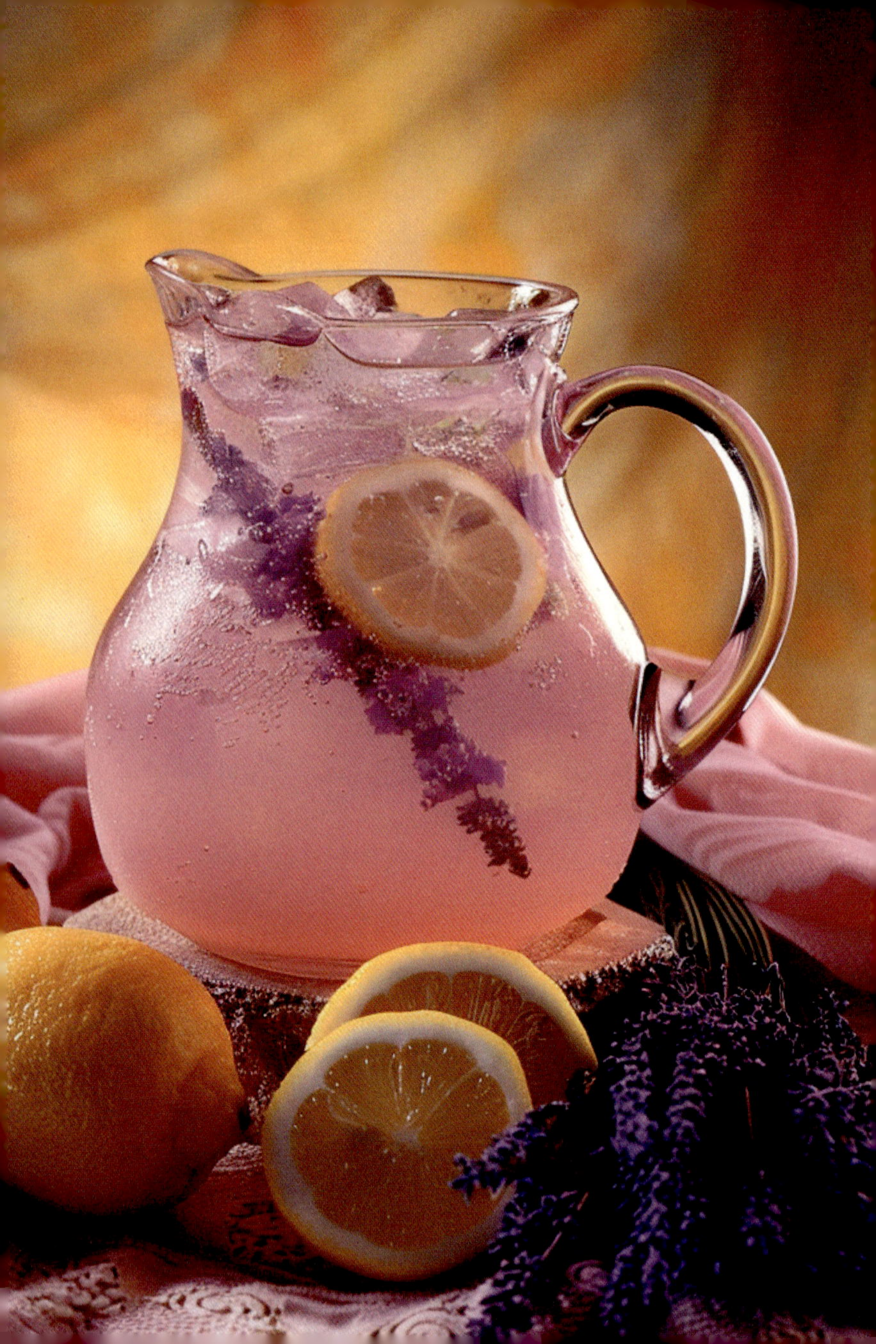

Azure Citrus Mixer

Inspired by Paul Stamets's Blue Juice, this mixer is loaded with bright citrus flavors, luscious red strawberries, and blackberries bursting with flavor. Combined with just enough sweetener—and some seltzer water to give it a little effervescence—you have yourself an easy to put together mixer perfect for sharing with a group during a long day in the sun (or the shade, inside, outside, up a tree, wherever you like). As with most of our recipes, we have steered away from using added sugar as a sweetener, but you can always do a quick swap if you prefer cane sugar or any other 1/1 sugar substitute.

Yield

Roughly 10 glasses

Dose

1.3 grams per serving

Ingredients

5 1/2 cups cold fresh water

2 1/2 cups Blue Juice (see page 101)

2 3/4 cups lemon juice

2 cups monk fruit sweetener

1 cup Empress 1908 Gin (Optional)

2 cups fresh strawberries, sliced

1 cup fresh blackberries

1 bottle of sugar-free seltzer water (set aside for later)

Ice

Preparation

Simple and quick, this will be done in a jiffy! In a large pitcher combine 5 1/2 cups of water, 2 cups of Blue Juice, lemon juice, and your gin. Next, add in the monk fruit sweetener and stir until fully dissolved. Now, add in the sliced strawberries and blackberries. Top this with ice and stir until chilled.

Serving

Grab some glasses (and fancy drink umbrellas) and fill them about halfway with ice. Pour in some of the mixer, until about 3/4 full, then top it all off with seltzer water for a little bubbly action. Share them with your mates and enjoy a refreshingly bright, tasty, little drink that will get you going on a hot day and open your mind to the possibilities of life!

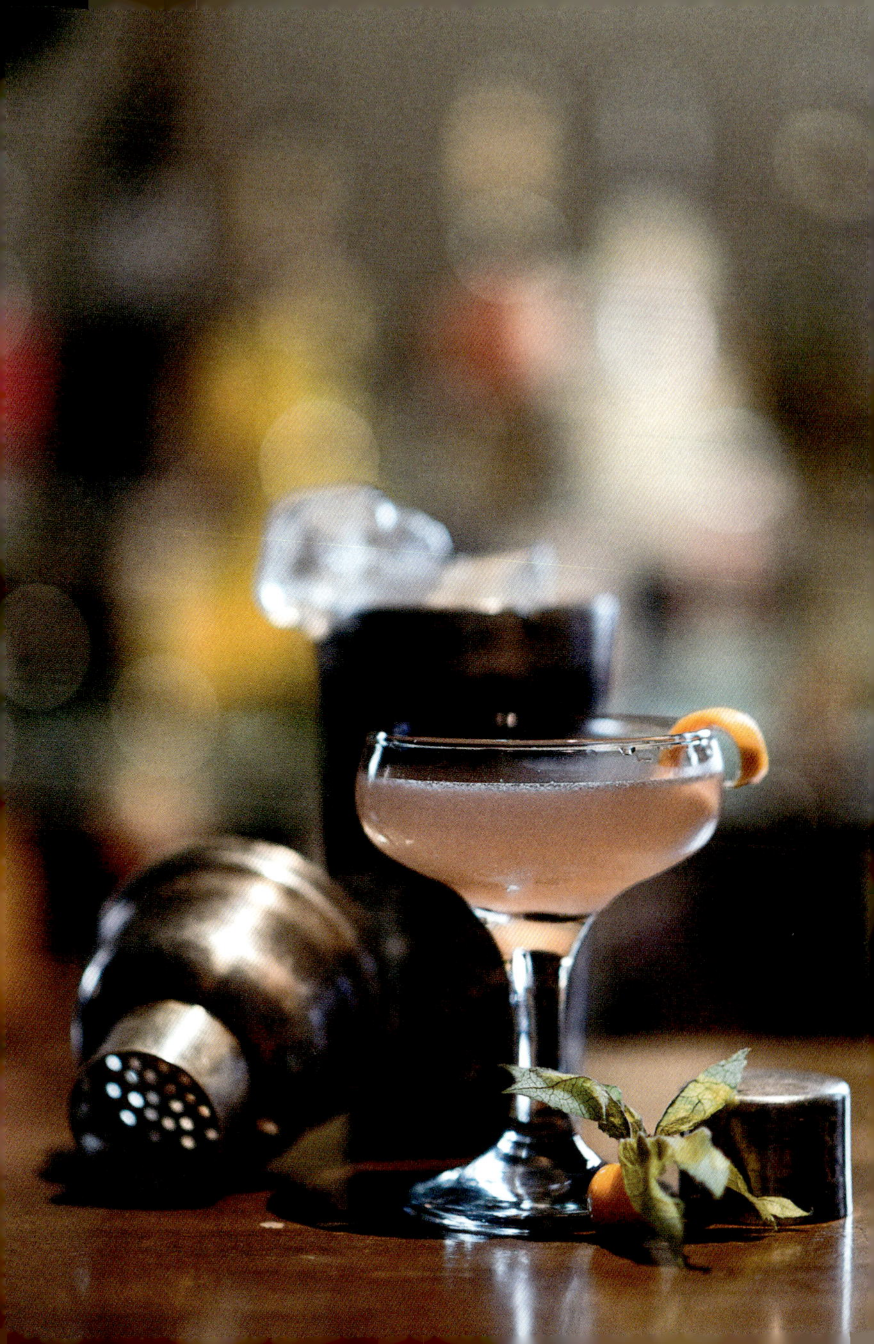

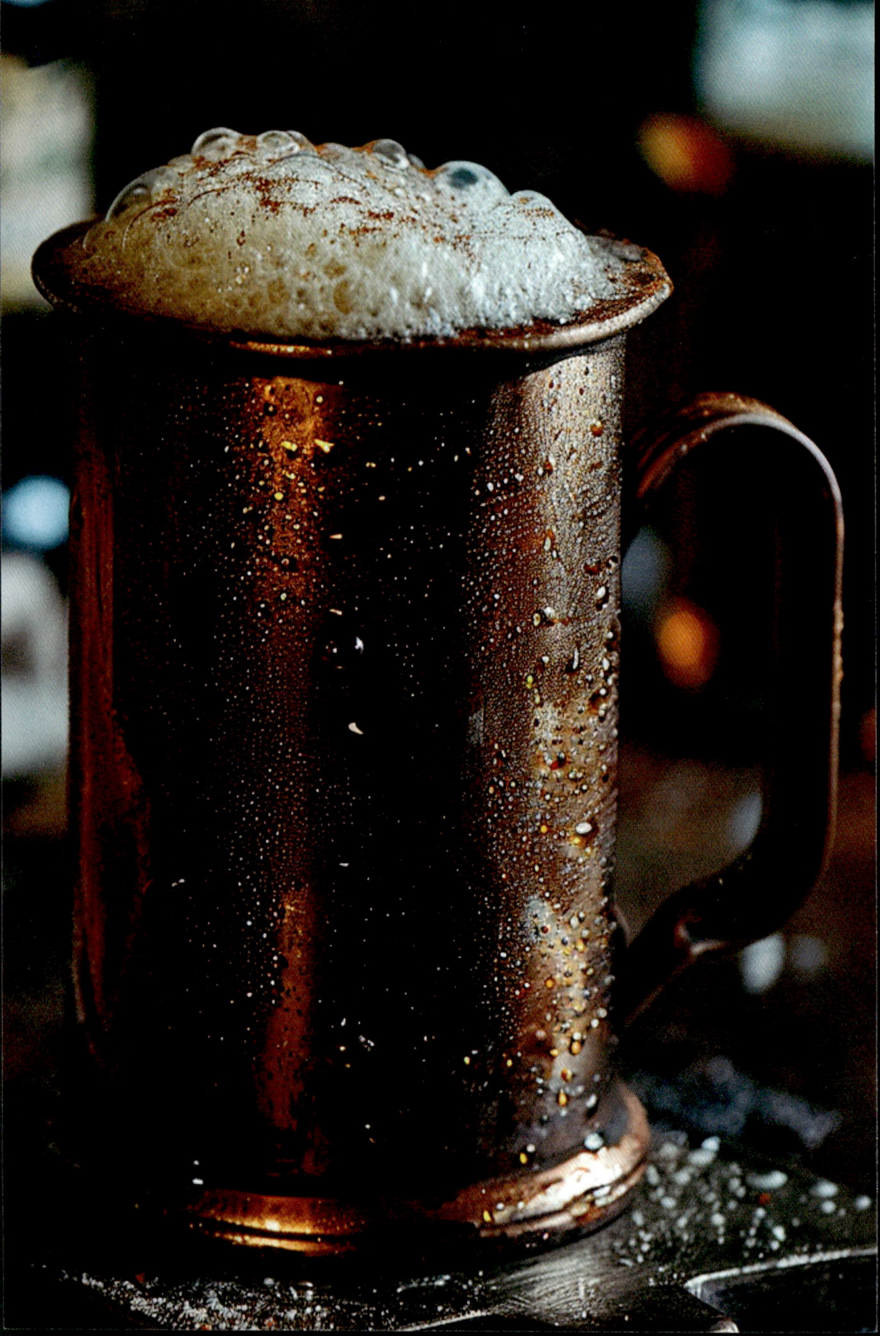

Cubensis, Root and Rye Cooler

I was inspired to create this unique cocktail after sharing a tall glass of Sassafras tea with my grandmother, who still goes out to harvest the roots herself on our family land in the Appalachian Mountains of Southwest Virginia. The tea's flavor profile is wonderfully complex and decidedly root beer-like for those that have never tried it. When mixed with good rye whiskey, a bit of Mushroom Elixir, and a dash of birch beer, flavors are earthy, fresh, and delightful. I find that it is the perfect medium for carrying you off on a journey of self-discovery, and it is my go-to drink when I want to simply mix, sip, and enjoy. Unfortunately, sassafras root is not widely available, so we have substituted it for sarsaparilla root which has a similar flavor profile.

Yield

1 serving

Dose

1 gram per serving

Ingredients

2 oz Organic Sarsaparilla Root Tea Concentrate (Chilled)

2 oz of rye whiskey

6 oz organic sugar-free birch beer (or root beer)

2 ml Mushroom Elixir (scale up or down as needed)

Sliced lemon for garnish

Note…

This recipe calls for a concentrated tea. To create the Sarsaparilla Root Tea concentrate, take 15 bags of any good Sarsaparilla Root Tea (we used Buddha Tea Organic Sarsaparilla Root Tea) brewed with 8 cups of water. This will create a potent tea concentrate. I wouldn't recommend drinking it—dilute it with three-parts fresh water to one-part concentrate. It's great to have on hand and saves time and space in the fridge.

Preparation

In a copper "Moscow Mule" style mug (it keeps the cocktail chilled longer and you get bonus fancy points), add in the tea concentrate, Mushroom Elixir, and rye whiskey. Give this a quick stir, and then add ice. Feel free to use frozen 1 oz Blue Juice cubes, but remember that it will change the dose. Top this off with the birch beer.

Serving

Squeeze in a bit of lemon juice from a nice fresh wedge, and then kick back and enjoy. This little mixer is great for a relaxing afternoon or a post meal aperitif. As always, it's best enjoyed with friends, so make a few, and happy journeys!

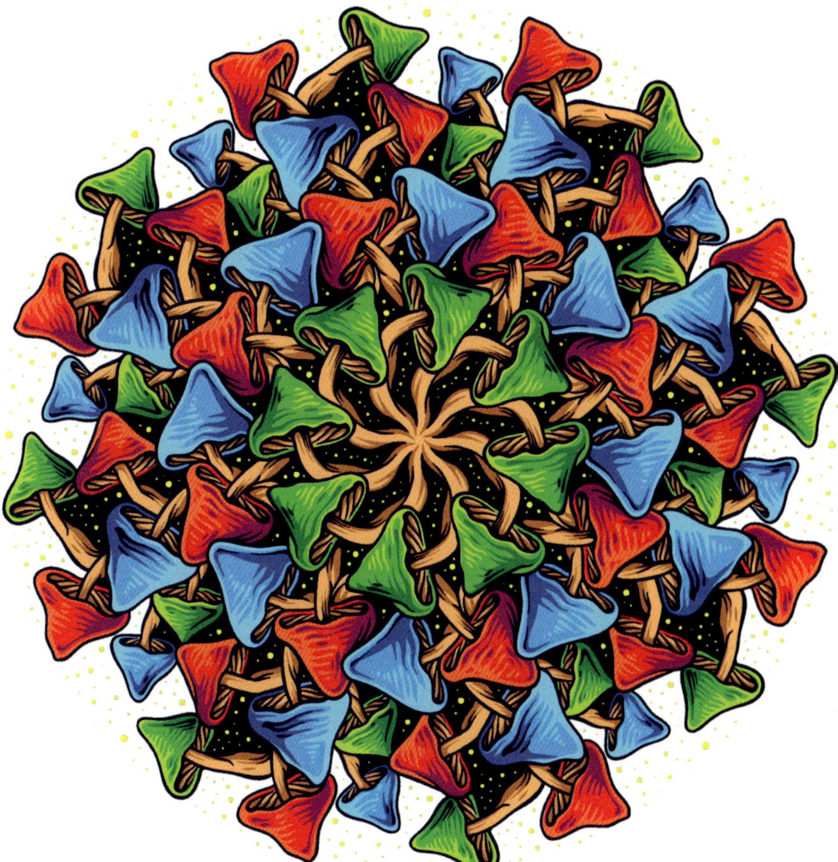

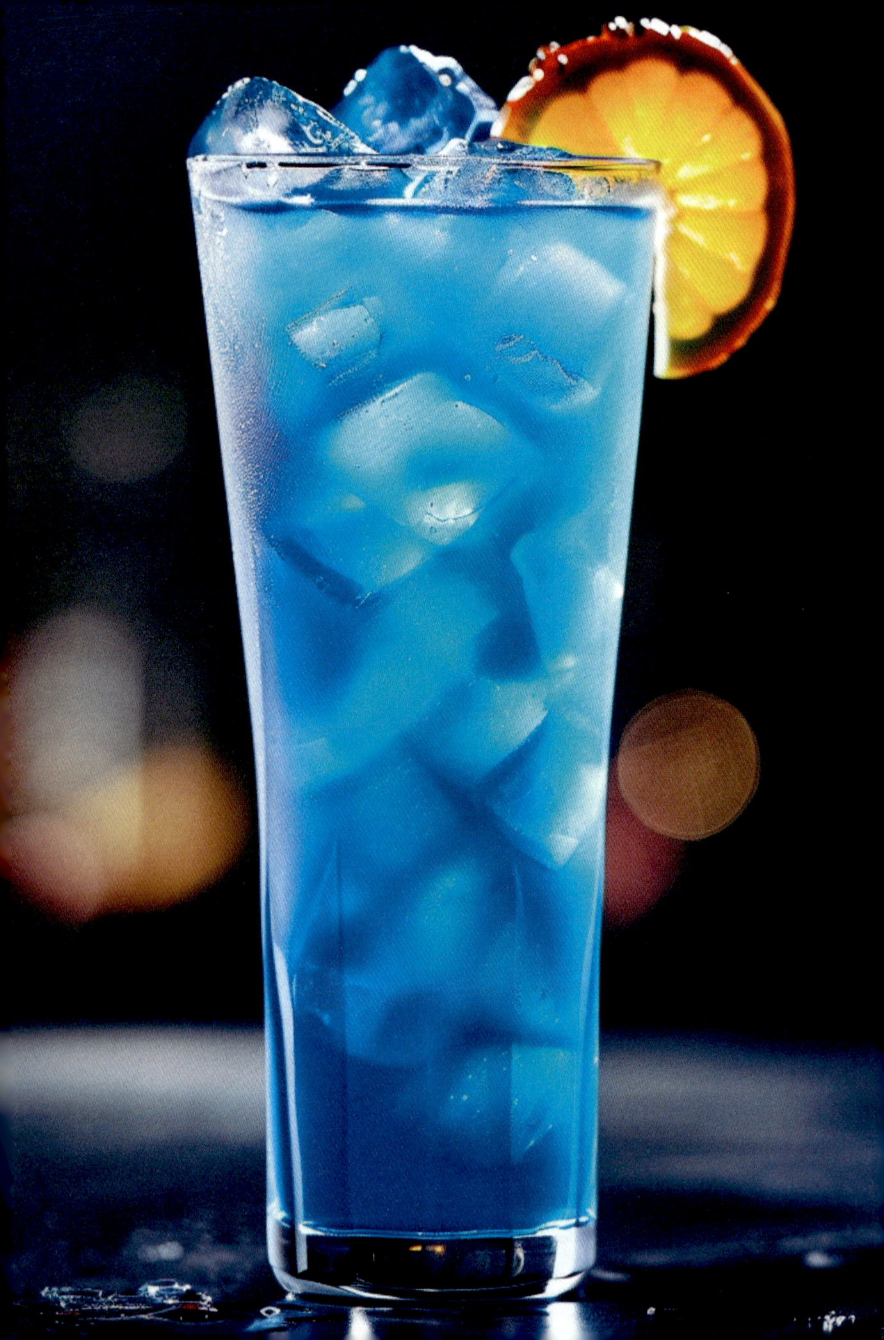

Elven Mana Potion

This is a fun one! We came up with the idea for this after making a pot of butterfly peaberry tea (which is naturally a deep emerald blue). I added in some Slivovitz Old Plum Brandy, Blue Juice, and purple Italian basil-infused ice cubes, plus a touch of lavender honey, to create a warm and complex potion that will take you to another world. My only warning is that the dosing with this particular drink is higher than some of our others (coming in at 1.3 grams per serving), so please use caution and be mindful of the power behind this amazing concoction. It is designed to yield two servings, so I suggest whipping it together with a trip partner.

Yield

2 servings

Dose

1.3 grams per serving

Ingredients

- *1/2 cup chilled butterfly peaberry tea*
- *1/2 bunch fresh Italian purple basil*
- *1 teaspoon lavender honey*
- *1 cup Blue Juice*
- *2 oz Slivovitz Old Plum Brandy*
- *3 drops Angostura Bitters*
- *Lemon twist for serving*

Preparation

Begin by preparing the peaberry tea as directed on the packaging. Once it's been brewed, sweeten the tea with lavender honey and allow it to cool in the refrigerator. While that chills, finely chop the basil, sprinkle this into your ice cube tray, and then add cold water to freeze.

Break time, sit back and relax for a while (or as I prefer, take a nap).

When your ice cubes are ready, grab the chilled peaberry tea and the ice cubes. In a cocktail mixer, combine the tea, Blue Juice, brandy, and bitters. Add in three or four cubes of regular, or Blue Juice, ice cubes and shake until cold. Strain into two chilled Cognac glasses over the basil infused ice.

Serving

Grab your glasses and a friend. Now take a thin slice of lemon peel and crush it to release the oil and acids. Throw this into your glass and watch the magic happen. This gorgeous potion demands slow sipping to maximize the enjoyment, so find your favorite gathering place, and allow your mind to wander through a garden of creativity and reflection.

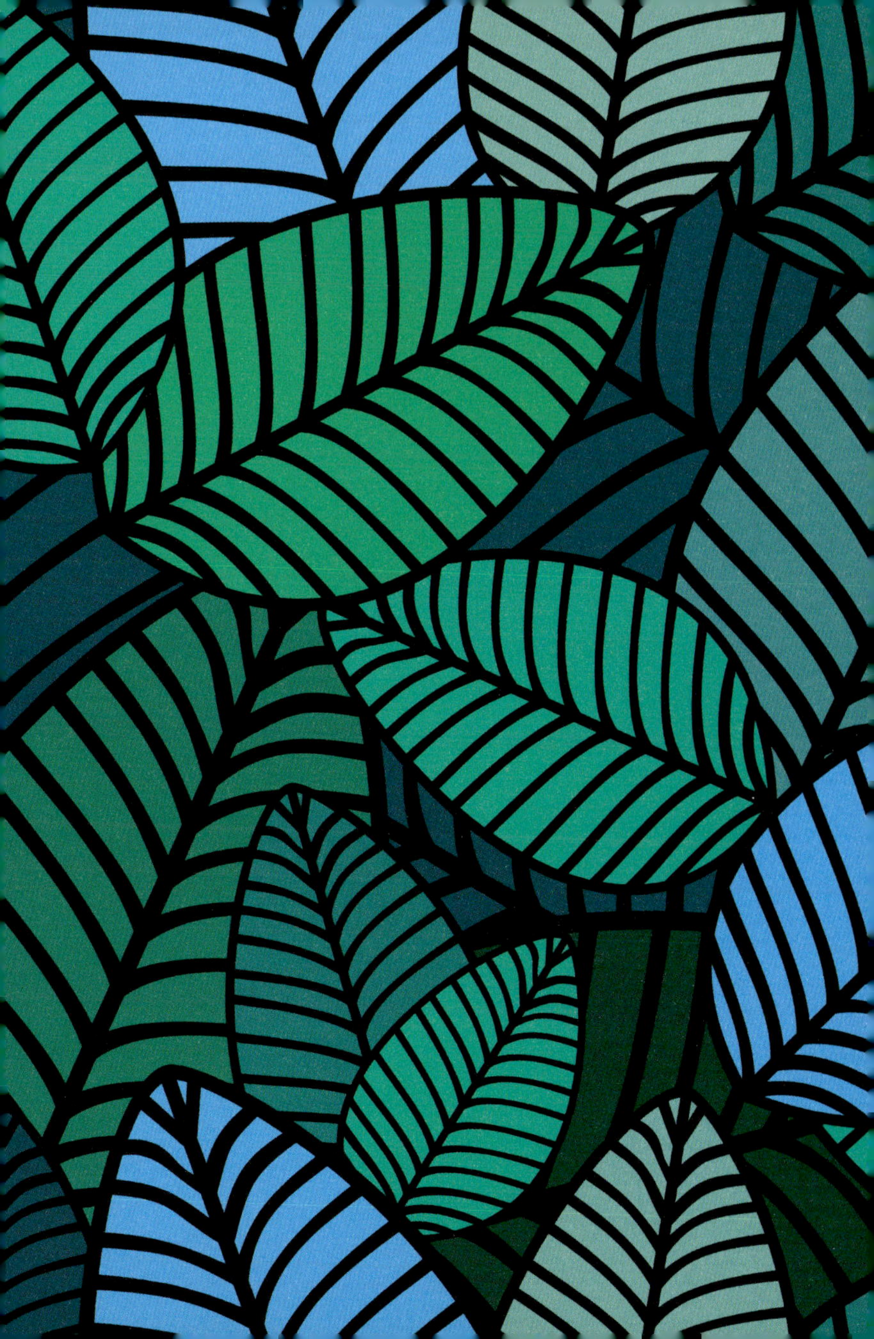

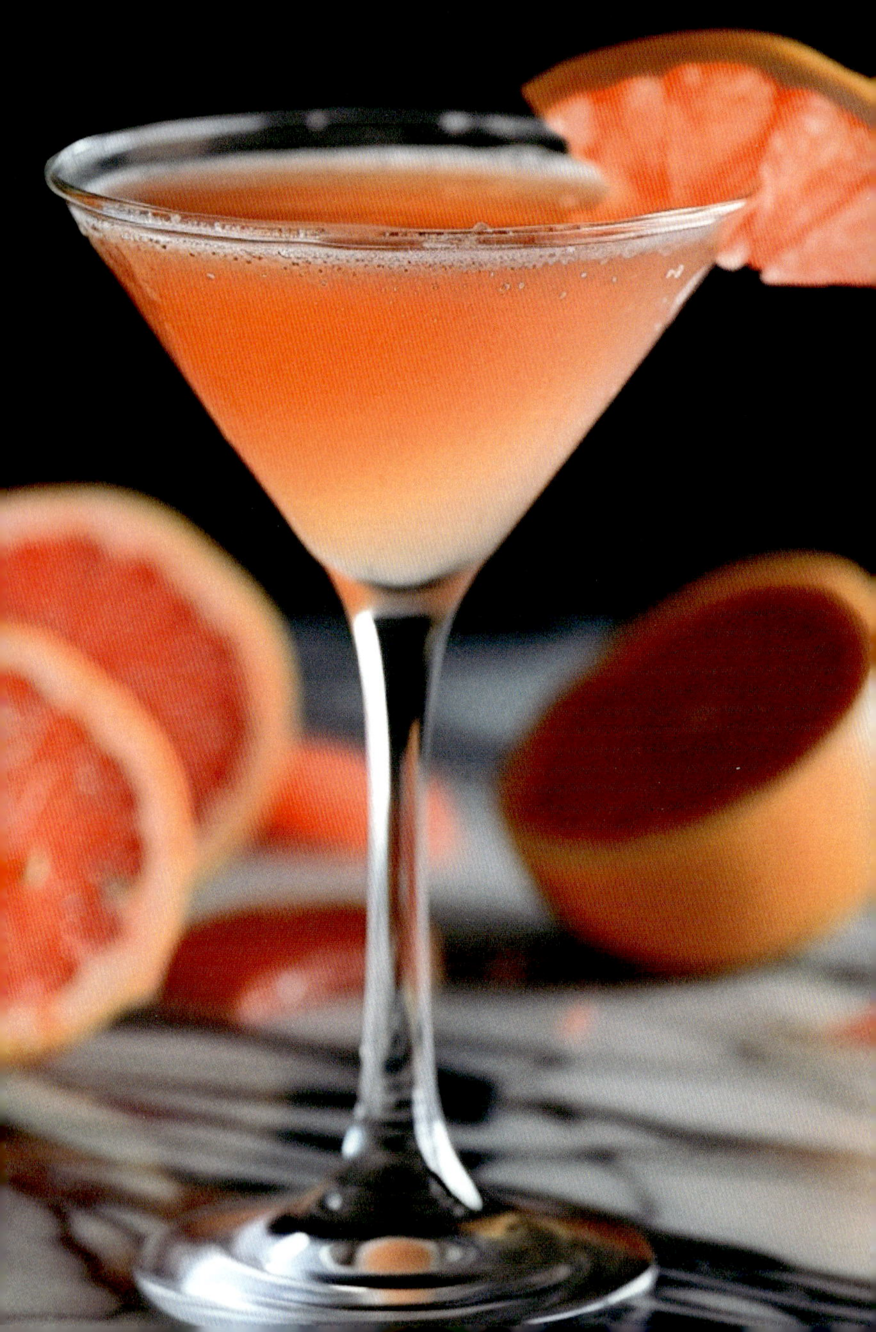

Dragon's Blood Martini

Stiffen your upper lip for this one, the Dragon's Blood martini is a strong, in-your-face drink charged with potent floral and fruit flavors that will take your taste buds for a spin. Tinto Red Premium Gin mixes with a dash of cranberry juice, and Foss Bjork Birch Liqueur, plus a little bit of dry vermouth, all held together by our Mushroom Elixir. The end result is a warm, spicy drink that will make you see dragons.

Yield

1 serving

Dose

1 gram per serving

Ingredients

1/2 oz dry vermouth

3 oz Tinto Red Premium Gin

2 oz Foss Bjork Birch Liqueur

2 oz cranberry juice

2 ml Mushroom Elixir

Preparation

Start by washing a cocktail shaker with the dry vermouth and pour out the excess (maybe into your mouth?). Fill the shaker about halfway with ice and then add the remaining ingredients, including the Mushroom Elixir, and shake the hell out of it (we want this ice cold). Once well-shaken, strain it into a martini glass.

Serving

This beautiful cocktail really stands out in a nice martini glass garnished with a few fresh, red berries (such as strawberries or cranberries) on a cocktail sword or toothpick. Make a few and share them, or kick back in your favorite lounger and prepare for your quest!

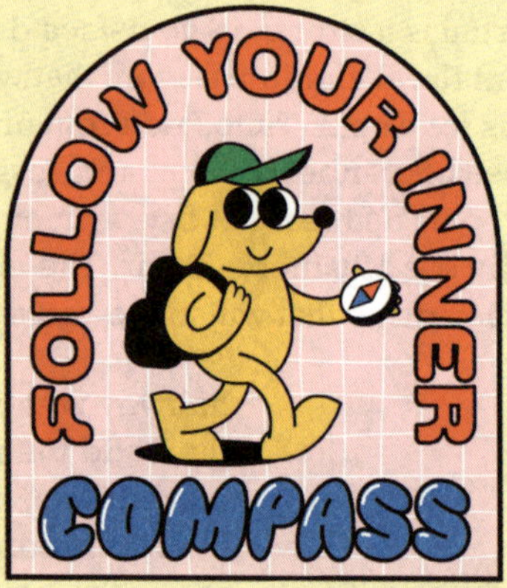
FOLLOW YOUR INNER
COMPASS

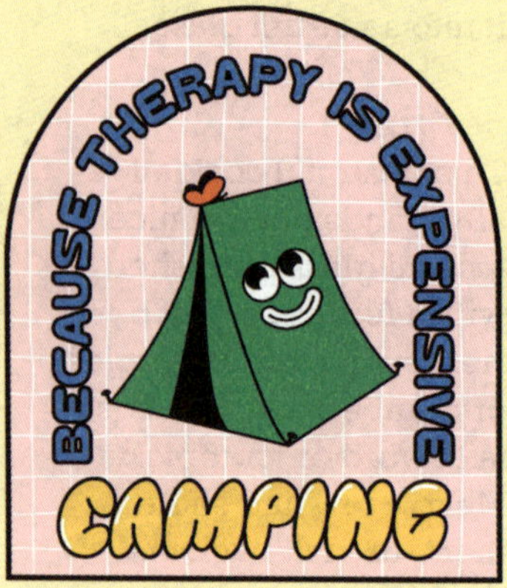
BECAUSE THERAPY IS EXPENSIVE
CAMPING

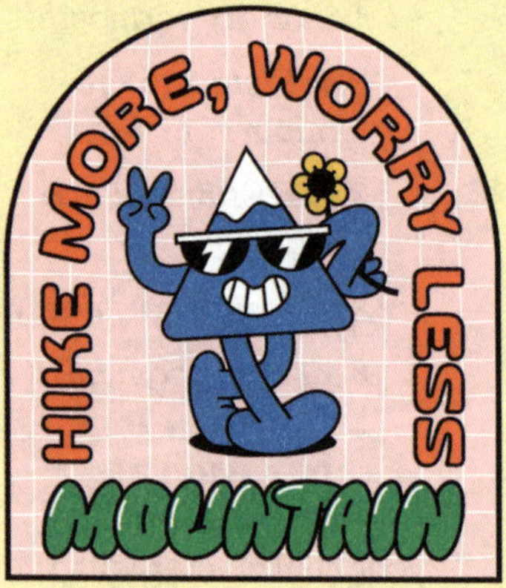
HIKE MORE, WORRY LESS
MOUNTAIN

RESOURCES

Works Cited

Akers, B.P., Ruiz, J.F., Piper, A. *et al.* A Prehistoric Mural in Spain Depicting Neurotropic *Psilocybe*

Mushrooms?. *Economic Botany* 65, 121–128 (2011). doi.org/10.1007/s12231-011-9152-5

Dutta V. Repression of death consciousness and the psychedelic trip. J Cancer Res Ther.

2012 Jul-Sep;8(3):336-42. doi: 10.4103/0973-1482.103509. PMID: 23174711.

Griffiths RR, Johnson MW, Carducci MA, Umbricht A, Richards WA, Richards BD, Cosimano

MP, Klinedinst MA. Psilocybin produces substantial and sustained decreases in

depression and anxiety in patients with life-threatening cancer: A randomized double-blind trial. J Psychopharmacol. 2016 Dec;30(12):1181-1197. doi: 10.1177/0269881116675513. PMID: 27909165; PMCID: PMC5367557.

Grof, Stanislav. *Psychology of the Future: Lessons from Modern Consciousness Research*. State University of New York Press, 2000.

Oak, Annie. *Manual of Psychedelic Support: A Practical Guide to Establishing and Facilitating Care Services... at Music Festivals and Other Events*. Multidisciplinary Assn For Psychedelic Studies, 2017.

Shroder, Tom. *Acid Test: LSD, Ecstasy, and the Power to Heal*. Plume, 2022.

Websites to Check Out

Beckley Foundation: Psychedelic Research and Drug Policy—beckleyfoundation.org

DanceSafe, a 501(c)3 public health organization promoting health and safety within the nightlife and electronic music community. Founded in the San Francisco Bay Area in 1998 by Emanuel Sferios, DanceSafe quickly grew into a national organization with chapters in cities across North America.—DanceSafe.org

TripSit's Guide to Drug Combinations—tripsit.me

Usona Institute—usonainstitute.org/research

The Vaults of Erowid—erowid.org/psychoactives

Vyrostek, Snowflake, Snowzilla Arts, illustrator of *Cooking with Magic Mushrooms*—https://snowzillaarts.com and facebook.com/SnowzillaArts/

Zendo Project: Psychedelic Harm Reduction—zendoproject.org

ABOUT THE AUTHOR

Originally from Bluefield, Virginia, author David Connell now resides in Colorado, drawing inspiration from the state's breathtaking landscapes and vibrant psychedelic culture.

David is a proud veteran of the United States Air Force, where he dedicated over a decade of active service as well as several years in the Air Force Reserves. His career spanned numerous deployments as part of the Air Force Special operations Command. These deployments took him to Afghanistan, Africa, the Middle East, and elsewhere. During his tenure, David also devoted time to volunteering at a military hospital, a decision motivated by a desire to contribute positively. However, the harrowing sights of young soldiers arriving with severe injuries, as well as his own experiences, deeply affected him, leaving a lasting emotional and psychological impact.

Transitioning back to civilian life proved challenging for David. The aftermath of his service was a tumultuous period marked by a struggle with severe depression, anxiety, traumatic brain injury, and PTSD, conditions for which he was heavily medicated on a regimen of VA-prescribed antidepressants. Facing a dark spiral of suicidal thoughts, David sought alternative healing methods. His journey towards recovery and self-discovery led him to the exploratory use of psilocybin mushrooms. This unconventional path provided David with a profound sense of relief and understanding, helping him navigate the complexities of his post-service trauma. Through his psychedelic experiences, David has found a renewed sense of purpose and a passion for sharing his story, contributing to the broader conversation on mental health, and the therapeutic potential of psychedelics.